175 Current Topics in Microbiology and Immunology

ADP-Ribosylating Toxins

Edited by K. Aktories

With 23 Figures and 4 Tables

Springer-Verlag
Berlin Heidelberg NewYork
London Paris Tokyo
Hong Kong Barcelona
Budapest

Professor Dr. Dr. KLAUS AKTORIES
Institut für Pharmakologie
und Toxikologie
der Universität des Saarlands
6650 Homburg/Saar, FRG

ISBN 3-540-54598-0 Springer-Verlag, Berlin Heidelberg New York
ISBN 0-387-54598-0 Springer-Verlag New York Berlin Heidelberg

Library of Congress Catalog Card Number 15-12910
Printed in Germany

Typesetting: Thomson Press (India) Ltd, New Delhi; Offsetprinting: Saladruck, Berlin; Bookbinding: Lüderitz & Bauer, Berlin.
23/3020-5 4 3 2 1 0 – Printed on acid-free paper.

Preface

ADP-ribosylating toxins have been the focus of intensive research for more than 30 years. Researchers from diverse fields of science have taken an interest in these bacterial toxins; they are studied, for example, by microbiologists, biochemists, cell biologists, and pharmacologists. There are two principal reasons for the broad and still growing interest in ADP-ribosylating toxins. First, insights into the structure and functions of the toxins might be the key to prevention and treatment of diseases caused by the toxin-producing infectious microorganisms. Second, the ADP-ribosylating toxins provide potent and often unique pharmacological tools for the study of the physiological functions of their target proteins. The latter is especially the case with cholera and pertussis toxins, which both modify the α-subunits of heterotrimeric G-proteins involved in signal transduction pathways. These toxins have proved invaluable in extending our basic understanding of the regulation of hormone-controlled signal transduction.

This volume provides a review and an update of recent studies on the basic properties of bacterial ADP-ribosylating toxins and/or exoenzymes. Our current knowledge of the cellular entry mechanisms of ADP-ribosylating toxins is reviewed by MADSHUS and STENMARK. WILSON and COLLIER then deal with recent insights into the enzyme mechanism and active site structure of diphtheria toxin and *Pseudomonas aeruginosa* exotoxin A, which modify elongation factor 2. Toxins which ADP-ribosylate heterotrimeric G-proteins involved in transmembrane signal transduction are the subject of the next two chapters. SERVENTI, MOSS and VAUGHAN describe the regulation of adenylate cyclase by cholera toxin and the enhancement of the cholera toxin-induced ADP-ribosylation by guanine nucleotide-binding proteins, the so-called ADP-ribosylation factors, and the review of pertussis toxin by GIERSCHIK lays emphasis on toxin structure–function relationship, toxin-G–protein interactions and the functional consequences of G-protein ADP-ribosylation. A chapter by AKTORIES, WILLE, and

JUST discusses recently described actin-ADP-ribosylating toxins such as *Clostridium botulinum* C2 toxin, *C. perfringens* iota toxin, and other iota-like toxins. Together with the mycotoxins cytochalasin and phalloidin, these ADP-ribosylating toxins appear to be important new tools with which to study the role of actin in various physiological processes. AKTORIES, MOHR, and KOCH deal with clostridial exoenzymes which modify small GTP-binding proteins. *C. botulinum* C3 ADP-ribosyltransferase, *C. limosum* exoenzyme, and their eukaryotic protein substrates Rho and Rac are discussed in detail. Last but not least, COBURN briefly reviews *P. aeruginosa* exoenzyme S. Much less is known about this ADP-ribosyltransferase and its eukaryotic substrates. Recent studies indicate that, again, small GTP-binding proteins (Ras proteins) are the preferred substrates of the enzyme.

This book offers an exciting and comprehensive account of recent developments in the field of ADP-ribosylating toxins and should inspire both further research in this area and the use of these toxins as tools in biological science.

K. AKTORIES

List of Contents

List of Contributors

(Their addresses can be found at the beginning of their respective chapters.)

This book is dedicated
to my mentor in toxinology,
Prof. Dr. Ernst Habermann

Entry of ADP-Ribosylating Toxins into Cells*

I. H. MADSHUS and H. STENMARK

Department of Biochemistry, Institute for Cancer Research at the Norwegian Radium Hospital, Montebello, N-0310 Oslo 3, Norway

* The authors were supported by the Norwegian Cancer Society.

Current Topics in Microbiology and Immunology, Vol. 175

1 Introduction

A number of bacterial toxins exert their action by ADP-ribosylating proteins essential for normal cellular function. In all cases known the substrate of these enzymes is either located free in the cytosol or associated with the cytoplasmic side of the plasma membrane. A key to understanding intoxication is therefore to understand how the toxins enter cells and get access to their cytoplasmic targets.

Most of the toxins can be divided functionally into two moieties, A and B. The A moiety carries the ADP-ribosyltransferase activity, whereas the B moiety mediates cellular uptake. The entry of ADP-ribosylating toxins into cells starts with their *binding to specific cell surface receptors*. At least in the cases of pseudomonas toxin and diphtheria toxin, the next step in the entry process involves *endocytic uptake*. Finally, a *membrane translocation* event is necessary to transport the enzymatically active moiety to the cytoplasmic side of the membrane.

In this review we will first describe the structure of the different ADP-ribosylating toxins and then sequentially discuss the binding, endocytosis (where relevant), and the membrane translocation step. We have chosen to deal with the different toxins individually. This review does not intend to cover the entry of *all* ADP-ribosylating toxins known, as the entry mechanisms of several toxins are to date unclear.

2 Structure of ADP-Ribosylating Toxins

2.1 Cholera Toxin and *Escherichia coli* Heat-Labile Toxins

Cholera toxin, an exotoxin produced by *Vibrio cholerae*, produces a massive noninflammatory secretory diarrhea when released in the small bowel, due to stimulation of adenylate cyclase (FINKELSTEIN 1973). The toxin is composed of five B subunits (12 kDa) that mediate the binding to cell surface receptors and one A subunit (27 kDa) which is responsible for the enzymatic effect of the toxin (Fig. 1; for review, see EIDELS et al. 1983). From evidence of a stoichiometry of AB_5 it was proposed that the A subunit lies on the central axis of a ring of B subunits (GILL 1977; LAI 1980; DWYER and BLOOMFIELD 1982). The A subunit is divided by proteolytic cleavage and chemical reduction into two fragments, A1 (22 kDa), which has catalytic activity, and A2 (5 kDa), presumed to mediate the interaction between A1 and the B subunits. Both cleavage and reduction seem to be required for catalytic activity (MEKALANOS et al. 1979).

Cholera toxin has been crystallized (SIGLER et al. 1977; MAULIK et al. 1988); however, the complete atomic structure has so far not been reported.

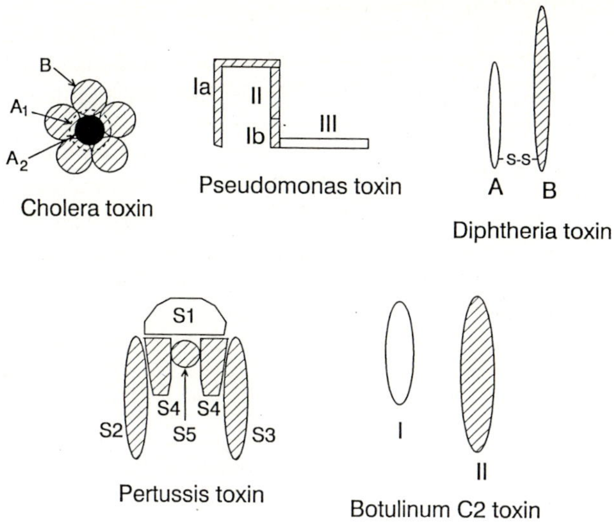

Fig. 1. Schematic structure of ADP-ribosylating toxins. The *hatched regions* represent putative binding/translocation parts of the molecules. The different molecules are not drawn to scale. Note that cholera toxin is shown in cross section (the A1 subunit is below the plane). See text for details

The *E. coli* heat-labile toxins resemble cholera toxin both in structure and in mode of action (for review, see HONDA et al. 1981; GEARY et al. 1982). Heat-labile enterotoxins are produced by enterotoxigenic *E. coli* and cause diarrhea in mammals. Several subtypes of heat-labile toxins have been reported (HONDA et al. 1981; GEARY et al. 1982; TSUJI et al. 1987). These toxins are, like cholera toxin, composed of two subunits, A and B, of which A has enzymatic activity, catalyzing the ADP-ribosylation of the stimulatory GTP-binding protein, thereby activating adenylate cyclase (HOLMGREN 1981). The B subunit is involved in binding to cellular receptors (see later). The crystal structure of a cholera toxin-related heat-labile enterotoxin from *E. coli* was quite recently reported, at a resolution of 2.3 Å (SIXMA et al. 1991).

2.2 *Pseudomonas aeruginosa* Exotoxin A

Pseudomonas toxin is one of the virulence factors produced by *Pseudomonas aeruginosa*. It is extremely toxic, having an LD_{50} of 0.2 μg upon intraperitoneal injection into mice (IGLEWSKI and SADOFF 1979). *Pseudomonas* toxin is toxic to eukaryotic cells because it specifically ADP-ribosylates a modified histidine (diphthamide) of elongation factor 2, a molecule involved in protein synthesis, thereby blocking peptide chain elongation (VAN NESS et al. 1980).

The mature form of the toxin is a single polypeptide chain of 613 amino acids. The crystal structure of the inactive form of exotoxin A was solved to

3.0-Å resolution (ALLURED et al. 1986). The amino acid sequence was reported by GRAY et al. (1984). Based on this sequence and the crystallographic data, ALLURED et al. (1986) proposed a model for the molecular structure of the toxin. The data provided support for a three domain model (see Fig. 1): domain I, comprising the N-terminal 252 amino acids (Ia) as well as amino acids 364–404 (Ib), is primarily composed of antiparallel beta sheets; domain II, comprising amino acids 253–364, is composed of six alpha helices, of which two appear to be surface-seeking and therefore likely to interact with hydrophobic membranes; and domain III, which was shown to contain the enzymatic activity of the molecule (GRAY et al. 1984), encompasses the C-terminal residues 405–613.

2.3 Diphtheria Toxin

Diphtheria toxin is secreted from *Corynebacterium diphtheriae* as a single polypeptide chain of 535 amino acid residues (58 kDa). The chain contains a highly trypsin-sensitive region (Arg-Val-Arg-Arg). Cleavage in this region ("nicking") is required for activity and yields two disulfide-linked fragments, A (21 kDa) and B (37 kDa) (Fig. 1; DRAZIN et al. 1971). The B fragment mediates receptor binding and membrane translocation (see below), whereas the A fragment is an ADP-ribosyltransferase that kills cells by inactivating elongation factor 2 (HONJO et al. 1968), in the same way as does *Pseudomonas* toxin.

The primary sequence of the toxin, deduced from its nucleotide sequence, has been determined (GREENFIELD et al. 1983; RATTI et al. 1983). By using an algorithm based on hydrophobic moment plot, EISENBERG et al. (1984) estimated the B fragment to contain one highly amphipathic alpha helix and four putative transmembrane segments. LAMBOTTE et al. (1980) noted that two putative alpha helices in the N-terminus of the B fragment exhibited significant sequence similarity to amphipathic alpha helices in the lipid-binding domain of human apolipoprotein A-I. The toxin has been crystallized (COLLIER et al. 1982), but so far no high-resolution structure has been interpreted from the X-ray diffraction data. There is significant amino acid sequence homology between the enzymic domain of diphtheria toxin and that of *Pseudomonas* toxin (CARROLL and COLLIER 1988), implying that these domains have diverged from a common ancestral protein.

2.4 Pertussis Toxin

Pertussis toxin is released into the surrounding medium by virulent *Bordetella pertussis*. The toxin is 105 kDa and consists of the following subunits: S1 (26 kDa), S2 (22 kDa), S3 (22 kDa), S4 (12 kDa), and S5 (12 kDa). It is composed of two S4 subunits and one copy of each of the other subunits (TAMURA et al. 1982). As is the case with other ADP-ribosylating toxins, pertussis toxin can be divided into an enzymatically active part (A), consisting of the S1 subunit, and a binding/translocation part (B), composed of two dimers (S2–S4 and S3–S4) which are joined by the S5 subunit (Fig. 1). Pertussis toxin is poorly soluble in aqueous buffers, due to the hydrophobicity of the B protomer (TAMURA et al. 1982). Sequencing of the pertussis toxin gene has revealed that it exists as an operon with the cistron order S1, S2, S4, S5, S3 (LOCHT and KEITH 1986; NICOSIA et al. 1986). All subunits contain leader sequences, indicating that they are individually secreted into the periplasmic space of the bacterium, where they are assembled. The S1 subunit, which ADP-ribosylates certain GTP-binding regulatory proteins (reviewed by MOSS and VAUGHAN 1988), exhibits N-terminal sequence similarity to subunit A of cholera toxin. Subunits S2 and S3 share 67% amino acid homology (LOCHT and KEITH 1986; NICOSIA et al. 1986), but do not complement each other (TAMURA et al. 1982).

2.5. Botulinum C2 Toxin

Botulinum C2 toxin is produced by certain strains of *Clostridium botulinum*. The toxin is cytotoxic and is not to be confused with botulinum neurotoxin. It is sometimes referred to as botulinum "binary" toxin, since it consists of two separate components (Fig. 1; OHISHI et al. 1980). Component I (50 kDa) ADP-ribosylates nonmuscle actin (AKTORIES et al. 1986; AKTORIES and WEGNER 1989), whereas component II (105 kDa) binds to cell surface receptors (OHISHI and MIYAKE 1985). For the toxin to be active, trypsinization of component II is required (OHISHI and MIYAKE 1985); this yields an 88-kDa fragment, which has the ability to bind component I. The trypsinized component II tends to oligomerize into a 365-kDa complex, and it is not clear yet whether it is the monomer or the oligomer that binds component I (OHISHI 1987).

3 Binding of ADP-Ribosylating Toxins to Cells

3.1 Cholera Toxin and *E. coli* Heat-Labile Toxins

3.1.1 Cellular Receptors

VAN HEYNIGEN et al. (1971) first observed that effects of cholera toxin on the gut were blocked by mixed gangliosides. The effect was later shown to be accounted for by GM_1 (galactosyl-*N*-acetyl-galactosaminyl-[*N*-acetylneuraminyl] galactosylglucosylceramide). Cholera toxin interacts with GM_1 when the ganglioside is in solution, incorporated into liposomes, or present on the surface of cells. Increased toxin binding was observed with cells and membranes enriched in GM_1. Also, when cells were treated with neuraminidase, thereby increasing the concentration of GM_1, increased functional cholera toxin binding was observed (for review, see EIDELS et al. 1983).

The nature of the receptors for heat-labile *E. coli* toxins is still inconclusive. Heat-labile enterotoxins have been demonstrated to bind to glycoprotein(s) on rat and human intestinal brush-border membranes not recognized by cholera toxin (HOLMGREN et al. 1982, 1985; GRIFFITHS et al. 1986). Like cholera toxin, heat-labile enterotoxins also bind to ganglioside GM_1 (HOLMGREN 1973; SVENNERHOLM and HOLMGREN 1978). Cholera toxin and heat-labile *E. coli* toxins form two antigenically distinct groups; cholera toxin and heat-labile *E. coli* toxins type I were shown to have other carbohydrate-binding specificities than heat-labile *E. coli* toxins type II (FUKUTA et al. 1988).

3.1.2 Receptor-Binding Domains

The B protomer, which is responsible for the binding of cholera toxin and heat-labile *E. coli* toxins to cellular receptors, consists of a noncovalent pentameric aggregate of identical polypeptide chains (GILL 1976a). The primary structure has been determined (LAI 1977; KUROSKY et al. 1977a; DALLAS and FALKOW 1980; LOCKMAN and KAPER 1983; MEKALANOS et al. 1983; YAMAMOTO and YOKOTA 1983; TSUJI et al. 1984). Sequence analyses of B subunits in several subtypes of heat-labile *E. coli* toxins and cholera toxins revealed that all of the B subunits are composed of 103 amino acids and the amino acid sequence homologies between different subtypes are more than 80% (LAI 1977; KUROSKY et al. 1977a, b; DALLAS and FALKOW 1980; LOCKMAN and KAPER 1983; MEKALANOS et al. 1983; YAMAMOTO and YOKOTA 1983; TSUJI et al. 1984, 1987; LEONG et al. 1985; TAKAO et al. 1985; YAMAMOTO et al. 1987). In these sequences a region from residue 48 to 74 from the N-terminus of the B-subunit is conserved among the toxins, implying a significance of this region in keeping the functional conformation (LOCKMAN and KAPER 1983; YAMAMOTO and YOKOTO 1983; FINKELSTEIN et al. 1987). The conserved region may contribute to immunogenicity and to binding to cellular receptors (JACOB et al. 1983, 1984), though conclusive evidence with respect to binding has not been presented (IIDA et al. 1989).

Physical studies of the B subunit have shown that binding of GM_1, but not related gangliosides, induces a shift in the emission spectrum maximum of cholera toxin from 342 to 330 nm (MULLIN et al. 1976). This shift reflects a conformational change affecting the single tryptophan residue of the B subunit (residue 88). DE WOLF et al. (1981) found that this tryptophan residue is located in a positively charged microenvironment near the GM_1 binding site. This finding was supported by LUDWIG et al. (1985) who studied the contributions of various amino acids to the structure and function of cholera toxin B by making chemical modifications. Possible effects on conformation were evaluated by reactivity to monoclonal antibodies directed towards conformational eptitopes. These authors suggest that the lysines are essential for receptor interaction in order to maintain the required electrostatic interaction and that one lysine residue resides close to the GM_1 binding site. Also, data were presented indicating an essential function for the intramolecular disulfide bond in the B subunits. Other amino acids of suggested importance for the binding are Arg-35, Arg-67, Arg-73 (DUFFY and LAI 1979; LUDWIG et al. 1985), Gly-33 (TSUJI et al. 1985), and Ala-64 (IIDA et al. 1989).

3.2 Pseudomonas Toxin

3.2.1 Cellular Receptors

Pseudomonas exotoxin A enters susceptible eukaryotic cells by binding to a specific, yet undefined, receptor in a saturable manner (MANHART et al. 1984; MIDDLEBROOK and DOORLAND 1984). There have been difficulties associated with measurements of binding of radiolabeled toxin to cells, because the proportion of toxin bound nonspecifically at low temperatures is quite high. Binding to paraformaldehyde-fixed mouse LM fibroblasts at 37 °C was saturable (K_d 5.4 n*M*), was reversible, and indicated ca. 100 000 binding sites per cell (MANHART et al. 1984).

Recently, a *Pseudomonas* toxin-binding glycoprotein of molecular weight greater than 300 000 Da was isolated from mouse LM cells (THOMPSON et al. 1991).

3.2.2 Receptor-Binding Regions

During the last couple of years the role of domain I of *Pseudomonas* toxin in receptor binding has been confirmed by several authors. From the crystallographic data it could be argued that the structure of domain I was suggestive of a ligand-binding structure (ALLURED et al. 1986). HWANG et al. (1987) found that molecules containing structural domain Ia blocked cytotoxic activity of intact *Pseudomonas* toxin on sensitive cells, whereas molecules lacking structural domain Ia and containing structural domains II, Ib, and III failed to block cytotoxicity. In agreement with this, GUIDI-RONTANI and COLLIER (1987) demonstrated concentration-dependent protection against authentic *Pseudomonas* toxin by mutant toxins. Only mutants containing all or most of domain I gave strong protection.

Treatment of *Pseudomonas* toxin with reagents reacting with lysine residues was shown to reduce cytotoxicity without changing the specific ADP-ribosylating activity. Since there are no lysine residues in domain II, this indicated that lysines in domain I could play a role in receptor recognition (PIRKER et al. 1985). In order to determine which lysine residues of domain I were involved in cell recognition, all 12 were changed (one by one) to glutamic acid by directed mutagenesis. Results from these experiments indicated that Lys-57 was residing in the receptor-binding part of domain I (JINNO et al. 1988). The same authors did deletion mutagenesis and claimed that amino acids 225–252 were important for binding, since the deletion mutants had strongly reduced liver toxicity. The conclusion that the above-mentioned residues reside in the binding region can be questioned, because no control experiments were performed to exclude introduction of conformational changes.

CHAUDRY et al. (1989) showed that insertion of a hexanucleotide encoding either Glu-Leu or Glu-Phe between amino acids 60–61 resulted in 99% reduction in cytotoxicity and that the mutant *Pseudomonas* toxin dissociated much faster from mouse LMTK$^-$ cells than did wild-type toxin. The location of the insert was within a major concavity on the surface of domain I, suggesting that this concavity is important for toxin-receptor interaction. The authors claim that the mutation in this case did not destabilize the conformation of the toxin. The possibility exists that insertion of the dipeptide may disrupt one or more of the three beta strands lining the surface of the concavity (WICK et al. 1990). Whether domain Ib has any role in receptor recognition is still unclear. Deletion of this region did not reduce the toxicity of a fusion protein of transforming growth factor alpha (TGF-α) and *Pseudomonas* toxin with deleted domain Ia (SIEGALL et al. 1989).

3.3 Diphtheria Toxin

3.3.1 Cellular Receptors

Cells derived from most animals (with the exceptions of mice and rats) are sensitive to diphtheria toxin. Since radiolabeled toxin exhibits extensive nonspecific binding to cells, it is difficult to demonstrate specific binding to cells with low receptor numbers. The first convincing demonstration of a diphtheria toxin receptor was presented by ITTELSON and GILL (1973), who showed competitive binding to HeLa cells. BOQUET and PAPPENHEIMER (1976) estimated the receptor number on HeLa cells to be about 4000 per cell, but the level of nonspecific binding was in this case 60%–90%. MIDDLEBROOK et al. (1978) studied specific binding of the toxin to Vero (monkey kidney) cells. These cells possess an exceptionally high number of receptors (about 10^5/cell). The authors calculated an association constant of 9×10^8 l/mol at 4° C. SCHAEFER et al. (1988) showed that the receptor numbers on Vero and Chinese hamster ovary-(CHO)-K1 cells were higher on cells grown at low density than on cells grown at high density. It is assumed that sensitivity to diphtheria toxin mainly depends on the number of cell surface receptors, although receptor-bearing mutant cell lines defective in toxin entry have been isolated (MERION et al. 1983; ROBBINS et al. 1983, 1984; MARNELL et al. 1984a; ROFF et al. 1986; KOHNO et al. 1987).

Several laboratories have attempted to identify the diphtheria toxin receptor. Trypsin treatment of cells inhibited toxin binding, suggesting that the receptor is a protein (MOEHRING and CRISPELL 1974; OLSNES et al. 1985). On the other hand, phospholipase C treatment of cells also apparently removed the receptors, indicating that the receptor may contain a phospholipid component (MOEHRING and CRISPELL 1974; OLSNES et al. 1985). Alternatively, interactions between the toxin and membrane lipids may be important for binding (LAMBOTTE et al. 1980; PAPINI et al. 1987). Permeant anions in the medium are required for binding as well as for translocation, and anion transport inhibitors strongly inhibit both processes. These findings have led to the proposal that the diphtheria toxin receptor may be an anion exchange protein (SANDVIG and OLSNES 1984, 1986). Protein kinase C agonists such as 12-*O*-tetradecanoyl-phorbol-13-acetate (TPA) apparently remove diphtheria toxin receptors (OLSNES et al. 1986), implying that protein phosphorylation may play a role in normal receptor function. Since different compounds such as phospholipase C, trypsin, anion transport inhibitors, and TPA all almost completely inhibit toxin binding, there is probably only *one* population of functional diphtheria toxin receptors.

The identification of the functional diphtheria toxin receptor has been hampered by the fact that the toxin apparently binds to a number of non-productive receptors. This was demonstrated by ROBLES et al. (1982), who identified a number of diphtheria toxin-binding glycoproteins from the membranes of sensitive Vero and CHO cells. It turned out that some of these proteins actually originated from the fetal calf serum used to supplement the medium (ROBLES et al. 1983; EIDELS et al. 1983).

In more recent studies, CIEPLAK et al. (1987) found that receptor-bound toxin on Vero and BS-C-1 cells could be crosslinked to the cell membranes, forming complexes of 70–80 kDa, thus indicating cross-linking to 10- to 20-kDa membrane components. In accordance with this, they also affinity-isolated 10- to 20-kDa proteins by first incubating surface-labeled Vero cells with diphtheria toxin, then lysing the cells, and subsequently immunoprecipitating lysate proteins with antibodies against the toxin.

MEKADA et al. (1988) isolated from crude membrane fractions of Vero and L cells an RNase-sensitive inhibitor of specific diphtheria toxin binding. The existence of such an inhibitor could partly explain the difficulties in identifying the receptor. To circumvent the problem with the inhibitor, these authors used the mutant toxin crm197 to identify a putative receptor. The mutant toxin does not bind the inhibitor and binds to cells with even higher affinity than does diphtheria toxin (MEKADA and UCHIDA 1985). Affinity isolation using crm197 yielded a protein of 14.5 kDa, present in Vero cells but not in resistant L cells.

ROLF et al. (1989) prepared anti-idiotypic antibodies against diphtheria toxoid, and found that these antibodies inhibited toxicity. The antibodies were found to react with a 15-kDa membrane component of Vero cells. The antibodies did not inhibit binding of the toxin to cells, but the authors suggested that the 15-kDa protein may nevertheless be the toxin receptor or a part of it.

At present the relationship between the 10- to 20-kDa proteins identified by CIEPLAK et al. (1987), the 14.5-kDa protein isolated by MEKADA et al. (1988), and the 15-kDa protein identified by ROLF et al. (1989) is not clear. It also remains to be established whether any of these proteins constitutes a *functional* diphtheria toxin receptor.

3.3.2 Receptor-Binding Regions

It was early appreciated that the B-fragment of diphtheria toxin is involved in receptor binding (DRAZIN et al. 1971; UCHIDA et al. 1972). Binding studies with crm197, a mutant with a single mutation in the A fragment, indicated that also the A fragment could be involved in binding, since the mutant toxin bound with *higher* affinity than did wild-type toxin (MEKADA and UCHIDA 1985). Later studies with in vitro translated B fragment have shown that also B fragment alone binds to diphtheria toxin receptors and that the affinity is higher than for full-length toxin (MCGILL et al. 1989). This raises the possibility that the B fragment is entirely responsible for receptor binding, and that association with A fragment, due to steric hindrance, decreases receptor affinity. In the case of crm197, the mutation in the A fragment could alter the conformation of this fragment, decreasing its steric hindrance of receptor binding. In agreement with this, only the "nicked" form of crm197 exhibited increased affinity, whereas nicking had virtually no effect on binding of wild-type toxin (MEKADA and UCHIDA 1985).

Another spontaneous mutant, crm45, which has a C-terminal deletion of 149 residues, did not bind to receptors, indicating that the C-terminal part of the toxin is involved in receptor binding (UCHIDA et al. 1972, 1973). This idea was supported by the finding that a mutant toxin lacking only the 50 C-terminal residues also was defective in receptor binding (MURPHY et al. 1986). Recently, ROLF et al. (1990) showed that a hydroxylamine cleavage product comprising the 53 C-terminal amino acid residues was able to compete with the toxin for receptor binding. Apparently, this peptide bound with lower affinity than did whole toxin. Conceivably, the primary receptor binding region of the toxin is located within this C-terminal peptide, but also other regions of the B fragment may be involved in strengthening the binding to cells. The N-terminal part of the B fragment may represent such a region, as deletion of the N-terminal 31 residues of the B fragment (containing one of the putative amphipathic regions) decreased its binding to cells (MCGILL et al. 1989). Possibly, the region in the C-terminus of the toxin binds to the (protein) receptor, whereas the N-terminal amphipathic helices enhance the membrane association by binding to phospholipid headgroups. A model in which diphtheria toxin binding to cells is mediated not only by a protein receptor but also by phospholipid interactions has been presented (PAPINI et al. 1987).

3.4 Pertussis Toxin

Pertussis toxin binds to cells via the B protomer (TAMURA et al. 1982). The toxin has lectin-like properties,since it agglutinates certain species of erythrocytes (ARAI and SATO 1976) and binds to glycoproteins containing N-linked oligosaccharides, such as haptoglobin (IRONS and MACLENNAN 1979) and fetuin (SEKURA et al.1983; ARMSTRONG et al. 1988). BRENNAN et al. (1988) demonstrated specific binding of the whole toxin as well as of the purified B protomer to a 165-kDa glycoprotein present in CHO cell membranes. Binding was abolished by sialidase treatment. The toxin did not bind to a mutant CHO line with defective processing of N-linked oligosaccharides. These authors found no evidence of pertussis toxin binding to gangliosides. Although the 165-kDa glycoprotein is a likely candidate for a productive pertussis toxin receptor, functional studies in support of this have so far not been presented.

3.5 Botulinum C2 Toxin

The receptor binding of the C2 toxin is mediated by component II (OHISHI and MIYAKE 1985). The receptor is not identified, but trypsinized as well as non-trypsinized component II have hemagglutinating properties (OHISHI 1987), suggesting that this component may exhibit lectin activity.

4 Endocytosis of Cholera Toxin, Pseudomonas Toxin, and Diphtheria Toxin

4.1 Cholera Toxin

Cholera toxin must penetrate the plasma membrane to gain access to its substrate, which is located on the inner surface of the membrane (FARFEL et al. 1979). The A subunit, which consists of two peptides linked by a disulfide bond, is involved in the activation of adenylate cyclase (GILL and KING 1975; GILL 1976b; MOSS and VAUGHAN 1977; CASSEL and PFEUFFER 1978; GILL and MEREN 1978). A1 catalyzes the transfer of ADP-ribose from NAD to subunits of the guanine nucleotide regulatory component of the adenylate cyclase system (CASSEL and PFEUFFER 1978; GILL and MEREN 1978). The modification leads to a persistent activation of the cyclase. In contrast to the rapid increase in cyclase activity obtained in membrane preparations (GILL and KING 1975; GILL 1976b), cholera toxin activates adenylate cyclase in intact cells only after a lag time of approximately 15 min (KIMBERG et al. 1971; GILL and KING 1975; BENNETT and CUATRECASAS 1975; FISHMAN 1980). During this delay the A subunit is translocated across the membrane and reduced to form A1. The generation of A1 from cholera toxin in intact cells has been related to the activation of adenylate cyclase (KASSIS et al. 1982).

Cholera toxin was reported to enter cells by endocytic uptake into the neuronal Golgi-endoplasmic reticulum-lysosome system (GERL) (JOSEPH et al. 1978). Cholera toxin covalently linked to horseradish peroxidase was found to be efficiently internalized into vesicles and cisternae of the GERL at 37 °C, but not at 4 °C. It was shown by MONTESANO et al. (1982) that in cultured liver cells noncoated membrane invaginations are involved in binding and internalization of cholera toxin. These findings raise the possibility that endocytosis of the toxin may be required for access of the A1 peptide to the cytoplasmic domain of the plasma membrane and subsequent activation of adenylate cyclase. However, conclusive experiments have not been performed with respect to requirements for endocytosis. Thus, no experiments in which the endocytosis was efficiently inhibited and the effect on activation of adenylate cyclase studied, have so far been reported. It is possible that cholera toxin could be translocated directly across the plasma membrane. However, in polarized cells the substrate is localized in the basolateral membrane, whereas the toxin binds to the apical surface. Accordingly, one might suspect that an endocytic event could be necessary to transport the toxin to the target membrane in such cells.

Janicot et al. (1991) recently concluded that endocytosis was required for activation of adenylate cyclase in liver cells based on the observation that a subcellular Golgi-endosomal fraction stimulated adenylate cyclase activity more rapidly than did the plasma membrane fraction.

4.2 *Pseudomonas* Toxin

In order for *Pseudomonas* toxin to exert its cell-killing activity, the enzymatic moiety must somehow be transported to the cytoplasm. The events occurring between toxin binding and the enzyme reaction in the cytoplasm are unclear, and considerably less is known about the entry mechanism for *Pseudomonas* toxin than for diphtheria toxin. It was demonstrated that, after binding to specific components on sensitive cells, *Pseudomonas* toxin moves rapidly into coated areas on the cell membrane. The toxin is subsequently internalized into endosomes and moves to lysosomes after passage through the Golgi region (Morris et al. 1983). The fact that lysosomotropic drugs protect cells against intoxication by *Pseudomonas* toxin (Fitzgerald et al. 1980; Sundan et al. 1984) indicates that *Pseudomonas* toxin enters the cytoplasm from an acidic intracellular compartment. Lowering the temperature to 19 °C afforded protection when the temperature transition was accomplished within 15 min of the original endocytic event, whereas methylamine was protective when added within the first 7 min (Morris and Saelinger 1986). This suggests that *Pseudomonas* toxin enters an acidic compartment before reaching a step blocked by shifting the temperature from 37 °C to 19 °C. There have been speculations that the productive entry of *Pseudomonas* toxin occurs from the Golgi complex, but conclusive evidence is still lacking.

The C-terminal sequence of *Pseudomonas* toxin (Arg-Glu-Asp-Leu-Lys) has some resemblance to the sequence responsible for retention of proteins in the endoplasmic reticulum, Lys-Asp-Glu-Leu (Munro and Pelham 1987), as pointed out by Chaudhary et al. (1990). Chaudhary et al. (1990) showed that C-terminal deletions or amino acid substitutions that did not affect ADP-ribosylation activity still produced nontoxic molecules and they suggested that a common factor may be involved in the intoxication of cells by *Pseudomonas* toxin and retention of proteins in the lumen of the endoplasmic reticulum. However, it remains to be investigated whether the Arg-Glu-Asp-Leu-Lys sequence of *Pseudomonas* toxin actually can replace the Lys-Asp-Glu-Leu sequence as an endoplasmic reticulum (ER) retention signal.

4.3 Diphtheria Toxin

Weak bases (Kim and Groman 1965; Leppla et al. 1980; Mekada et al. 1981) and ionophores (Marnell et al. 1982) that increase the pH of intracellular vesicles were shown to protect cells against diphtheria toxin, suggesting that the toxin has to be endocytosed and reach an acidic intracellular vesicle for intoxication to occur. Electron microscopic studies with biotin-labeled diphtheria toxin visualized via avidin gold have indicated that diphtheria toxin molecules bound to Vero cells are endocytosed via coated pits. Apparently, only a minor fraction of the bound toxin is endocytosed rapidly (Morris et al. 1985). When endocytosis from coated pits was inhibited (Moya et al. 1985) cytotoxicity was blocked, consistent with a requirement of endocytic uptake for intoxication to occur.

When fusion between endocytic vesicles and the Golgi apparatus or lysosomes was inhibited at low temperature, intoxication still occurred (Marnell et al. 1984b; Sandvig et al. 1984). It therefore appears that diphtheria toxin enters the cytosol from acidic *endosomes*. Entry from endosomes is further evidenced by electron microscopy data (Morris et al. 1985).

5 Membrane Translocation of ADP-Ribosylating Toxins

5.1 Cholera Toxin

Different mechanisms for membrane insertion and translocation of the enzymatically active A1 fragment of cholera toxin have been proposed. A mechanism where surface-binding induces conformational changes in the B protomer, thereby creating a hydrophilic channel through which A1 can freely diffuse, was proposed by Gill (1976a). In accordance with this, cholera toxin was shown capable of forming cation-selective channels in bilayers containing the ganglioside GM_1 (Tosteson and Tosteston 1978).

Data suggesting preferential insertion of the A1 peptide into the lipid membrane were obtained from a model viral system (Wisnieski and Bramhall 1981). This correlates with the finding that A1 is hydrophobic in nature and tends to form aggregates (Tomasi et al. 1978). Wisnieski and Bramhall (1981) used the photoactivatable glycolipid probe 12-(4-azido-2-nitrophenyl)-stearoyl [1-^{14}C]-glucosamine (12-APS-GlcN). This probe spontaneously inserts into membranes and labels proteins within the outer monolayer of Newcastle disease virus, which is rich in GM_1 and therefore can bind cholera toxin. When toxin bound to the glycolipid probe-virus complex, A1 was rapidly labeled at 37 °C, but not at 4 °C. Also, there was essentially no labeling of the B subunits. This supports a model in which A1 does not enter through the channel formed by the B protomer.

TOMASI and MONTECUCCO (1981) found that when cholera toxin bound to liposomes containing GM_1, the B subunits were labeled by shallow-inserting photoreactive probes while *none* of the subunits were labeled by deeply inserted probes. This argues against spontaneous insertion of the A subunit into the membrane. The authors observed that after reduction of the disulfide bridge between A1 and A2, A1 was intensely labeled by photoreactive probes located deeply in the membrane. It thus seems that reduction of the toxin is a prerequisite for insertion of A1 into the membrane. The discrepancy between these results and the results reported by WISNIESKY and BRAMHALL (1981) could be explained by the possibility that there are free sulfhydryl groups in the membrane of Newcastle disease virus (PATZER et al. 1979) capable of reducing the disulfide bridge in the toxin.

Recently, the three-dimensional structure of cholera toxin penetrating a lipid membrane was obtained from two-dimensional crystals of cholera toxin bound to receptors in a lipid membrane. X-ray analysis revealed a ring of five B subunits on the membrane surface, with one-third of the A subunit occupying the center of the ring (RIBI et al. 1988). Cleavage of the disulfide bond in the A subunit was observed to cause a major conformational change, with the A subunit exiting from the B ring. The B oligomer and the A2 fragment were left behind, bound to the membrane surface, and essentially unaffected by the movement of A1. This report indicates a two-stage membrane penetration by A1, the first one occurring before reduction and the second one after. Perturbation of lipid packing and membrane penetration driven by GM_1 binding may explain the capacity of the A1 fragment to enter the hydrophobic interior of a membrane (RIBI et al. 1988).

The reduction of the disulfide bond in the A subunit seems to be an absolute requirement for complete membrane insertion/translocation by A1. This process could in principle be performed either on the external face of the plasma membrane by thiol protein disulfide interchange (MOSS et al. 1980) or at the cytoplasmic face by intracellular reducing agents such as glutathione.

5.2 *Pseudomonas* Toxin

As lysosomotropic drugs protect cells against intoxication by *Pseudomonas* toxin, low pH is probably at some point involved in the entry process. It has been shown by several authors that *Pseudomonas* toxin changes conformation upon exposure to low pH. FARAHBAKHSH et al. (1987) reported that the intrinsic fluorescence of *Pseudomonas* toxin is strongly dependent on pH, decreasing between pH 7.4 and 4.0. The changes were reversible and indicated exposure of hydrophobic surfaces. It was also shown that at low pH *Pseudomonas* toxin binds Triton X-114, again indicating exposure of hydrophobic regions (SANDVIG and MOSKAUG 1987). The Triton binding was induced at pH below 4. Recently, JIANG and LONDON (1990) reported that two distinct conformations exist at low pH. An intermediate low-pH state dominates at pH 3.7–5.4 and is distinguished by blue-shifted fluorescence and weak or no hydrophobicity. The second low pH state is dominant below pH 3.7 and is characterized by red-shifted fluorescence and strong hydrophobicity. The second state appears to be like a denatured state, and in this state *Pseudomonas* toxin strongly binds detergent micelles and binds and inserts into model membranes (JIANG and LONDON 1990). Therefore, denaturation-like conformational changes appear to play an important role in membrane insertion. The pH of the transition to a membrane-inserting state is influenced by the composition of the model membranes and is close to pH 5 in the presence of vesicles containing a phosphatidylglycerol/phosphatidylcholine mixture (JIANG and LONDON 1990).

Domain II of *Pseudomonas* toxin has been suggested to be important for the insertion/translocation process. No long stretches of hydrophobic amino acids (as found in diphtheria toxin) can be found in *Pseudomonas* toxin. However, it would be sterically feasible for the helices of domain II, protruding from the top of the molecule, to undergo a significant conformational change and to insert into and disrupt a phospholipid bilayer (ALLURED et al. 1986). The binding to Triton X-114 of the three domains of *Pseudomonas* toxin as a function of pH was investigated in order to study whether the increased Triton binding at low pH was due to a global change in the toxin or due to a change within a particular domain. Results showed that all the truncated toxin proteins (consisting of different domains) displayed a similar pH-dependent entry into the detergent phase as native toxin, with a transition point of 4.2 for *Pseudomonas* toxin and 4.4–4.5 for the truncated toxins (IDZIOREK et al. 1990). These results suggest that upon acidification *Pseudomonas* toxin becomes globally hydrophobic and is converted into a translocation-competent form.

To further localize the domain responsible for membrane translocation, various deletions and mutations of the gene encoding *Pseudomonas* toxin were performed. Toxin with an N-terminal deletion of domain II exhibited both binding activity and ADP-ribosylation activity, yet the deletion mutant was nontoxic to sensitive cells (HWANG et al. 1987). Fusion proteins of TGF-α and domain II and III of *Pseudomonas* toxin (PE40) were toxic to cells with receptors for epidermal growth factor (EGF). In contrast, when large portions of the N-terminal or C-terminal end of domain II were deleted, the resulting proteins were practically nontoxic. These molecules bound to EGF receptors and had ADP-ribosylating activity (SIEGALL et al. 1989). Furthermore, when the disulfide bridge within domain II was removed by replacing Cys-265 and Cys-287 by serine, the cytotoxicity was reduced, presumably due to less efficient translocation (MADSHUS and COLLIER 1989). The mutant toxin lacking the disulfide bridge in domain II was much less stable than wild-type toxin, and the lower cytotoxicity could be due to accelerated intracellular degradation or abortive, premature membrane insertion (MADSHUS and COLLIER 1989). In summary, most results indicate that domain II is involved in membrane translocation. However, since manipulations of domain II seem to easily perturb the stability of the protein, negative results with respect to cytotoxicity are not direct evidence that domain II possesses translocation activity. Structural genes encoding C-terminal fragments of *Pseudomonas* toxin have been cloned and expressed, and shown to be enzymatically active (GRAY et al. 1984). Proteolytic processing of *Pseudomonas* toxin has been suggested to take place inside an intracellular organelle and could be a prerequisite for efficient translocation of the enzymatic domain to the cytosol.

For *Pseudomonas* toxin direct and good translocation assays are still lacking, even if liposome studies have been useful to clarify certain aspects of the insertion/translocation process (FARAHBAKHSH et al. 1986). This is in contrast to diphtheria toxin, where entry of surface-bound toxin can be induced by incubating the cells at low pH and where the fate of correctly inserted radiolabeled toxin can be studied (see below).

5.3 Diphtheria Toxin

5.3.1 Conformational Alterations at Low pH

The last step in the entry pathway of diphtheria toxin involves its passage from acidic endosomes into the cytoplasm (for a recent review, see SANDVIG and OLSNES 1991). Diphtheria toxin is readily water-soluble at neutral pH, and consequently not suited to insert into membranes under neutral conditions. However, there is ample evidence that the low pH encountered in endosomes imposes on the toxin significant conformational changes to make the toxin hydrophobic. At pH below 5.3 the toxin binds the detergent Triton X-100 (SANDVIG and OLSNES 1981). Fluorescence intensity and circular dichroism measurements (BLEWITT et al. 1984, 1985a, b) likewise suggested cooperative, denaturation-like changes taking place at low pH, with internally buried tryptophan residues apparently becoming more exposed.

It has been suggested that the A-fragment may enter the cytosol in an unfolded state through an aqueous channel formed by the B fragment (KAGAN et al. 1981). However, data obtained by several groups show little evidence of extensive A-fragment unfolding and indicate that not only the hydrophobic B fragment, but also the more hydrophilic A fragment, may associate with lipids at low pH (HU and HOLMES 1984; MONTECUCCO et al. 1985; ZHAO and LONDON 1986, 1988; CABIAUX et al. 1989). This implies that even the A fragment makes contact with membrane lipids during translocation. The N-terminal region of the B fragment, containing putative amphipathic helices (LAMBOTTE et al. 1980), became trypsin sensitive at low pH (DUMONT and RICHARDS 1988). It was proposed that the amphipathic regions may become exposed at low pH, possibly forming a membrane-seeking structure.

CABIAUX et al. (1989) employed infrared spectroscopy to evaluate the conformation of diphtheria toxin at pH 7.3 and pH 4.0 in the presence of acidic liposomes. They found that a cyanogen bromide fragment containing the hydrophobic middle region of the B fragment exhibited an increase in alpha helix content at low pH. Circular dichroism measurements indicated that the alpha helices were oriented parallel to the membrane lipids, thus representing a transmembrane structure. By contrast, another cyanogen bromide fragment containing the putative amphipathic regions in the N-terminus of the B-fragment appeared to adopt an increase in beta sheet configuration with strengthened hydrogen bonds at low pH, together with a large increase in the ability to bind lipids. Apparently, the beta sheets were perpendicular to the membrane lipids, in agreement with the suggestion that the amphipathic regions may react with the upper surface of the lipid bilayer (LAMBOTTE et al. 1980; DUMONT and RICHARDS 1988). In contrast to the isolated B fragment, the A fragment exhibited extensive conformational changes at low pH, with a significant decrease in alpha helix content and a concomitant increase in beta sheet content.

5.3.2 Translocation Directly Across the Plasma Membrane

Because it is difficult to manipulate the conditions on either side of the endosomal membrane in a controlled manner, it is a great advantage that translocation of diphtheria toxin can be induced directly across the plasma membrane by exposing cells with surface-bound toxin to low pH (DRAPER and SIMON 1980; SANDVIG and OLSNES 1980). This also has the advantage of obtaining a synchronized translocation event. It is assumed that the low pH-induced translocation across the plasma membrane resembles that taking place across the endosomal membrane in vivo.

Studies by SANDVIG et al. (1986) have shown that translocation does not take place when the cytosol is acidified, and that a *proton gradient* of at least one pH unit is required. The role of the low pH therefore seems to be dual: (1) The toxin changes conformation and exposes hydrophobic regions at low pH. (2) A proton-motive force appears necessary to drive the A fragment across the membrane. HUDSON et al. (1988) reported that the membrane potential also seemed to be important as a driving force for translocation of fragment A. However, this is in contradiction to findings by SANDVIG et al. (1986).

MOSKAUG et al. (1987, 1988) studied translocation across the plasma membrane directly at low pH by tracing radiolabeled diphtheria toxin bound to Vero cells. The disulfide bridge linking fragments A and B was reduced during translocation, presumably when exposed to the reducing conditions in the cytosol. Whereas the whole A-fragment was translocated to the cytosol and thereby shielded from extracellularly added proteases, only a part of the B fragment (25 kDa out of 37 kDa) was protease protected. In contrast to the A fragment, the 25-kDa B-fragment-derived polypeptide was membrane associated, presumably as a result of insertion in the plasma membrane. Interestingly, the 25-kDa polypeptide (but not the A-fragment) became protease protected as a response to low pH, even in the *absence* of a proton gradient, indicating that a proton-motive force is necessary to drive the A fragment across the membrane, but not for membrane insertion of the B fragment. The 25-kDa polypeptide extends from around residue 300 and to the very C-terminus of the toxin (MOSKAUG et al. 1991).

MOSKAUG et al. (1987) also observed that only 5%–10% of the A fragment associated with the cells was actually translocated at low pH. This agrees with earlier results (MOYNIHAN and PAPPENHEIMER 1981), which indicated that only a minor fraction of the bound toxin molecules ever reach the cytosol.

5.3.3 Diphtheria Toxin-Induced Ion Channels

Concomitantly with low pH-induced translocation across the plasma membrane, cation-selective channels are formed (PAPINI et al. 1988; SANDVIG and OLSNES 1988). Diphtheria toxin also forms cation-selective channels in artificial lipid membranes (KAGAN et al. 1981; DONOVAN et al. 1981) and lesions in the inner membrane of *E. coli* (O' KEEFE and COLLIER 1989). The channels formed in the plasma membrane and in model membranes have the same requirements for a transmembrane pH gradient and they have the same ion selectivity. However, it is to date not clear whether the channels studied in these different systems are identical. Electrophysiological measurements on whole cells treated with diphtheria toxin and low pH could clarify this issue.

The B-fragment alone can form channels in the plasma membrane with the same characteristics as those formed by the whole toxin, but with a 100-fold higher efficiency on a concentration basis (STENMARK et al. 1989). The increased efficiency can only partly be explained by a higher affinity for the receptors (McGILL et al. 1989). Apparently, the presence of the A fragment inhibits channel formation by the B fragment, either by plugging the channel or by interfering with interactions between the B fragment and the membrane.

PAPINI et al. (1988) showed that a translocation-incompetent mutant, crm1001, did not make channels. Likewise, our unpublished results indicate so far that mutants with defective channel formation invariably exhibit defective membrane translocation. Consequently, there appears to be a close interrelationship between the two events, even if the idea of A fragment translocation through a channel formed by the B fragment is no longer favored (see above). The channels stay open for several minutes (PAPINI et al. 1988; SANDVIG and OLSNES 1988; STENMARK et al. 1989), whereas A-fragment translocation is complete within 20 s at 37 °C (SANDVIG and OLSNES 1981). However, it is still not clear whether channel formation is a prerequisite for membrane translocation, or vice versa.

5.4 Pertussis Toxin

MONTECUCCO et al. (1986) studied the interaction of pertussis toxin with lipid micelles containing trace amounts of photoactivatable probes. Their results indicated that the S2 and S3 subunits (see Fig. 1) inserted deeply into lipid bilayers, whereas the S4 subunits exhibited a more shallow insertion. The S1 and S5 subunits were not found to react with the membrane probes. The results are consistent with the strong hydrophobicity of subunits S2 and S3 (LOCHT and KEITH 1986; NICOSIA et al. 1986), and indicate that membrane insertion of these subunits may be important in facilitating membrane translocation of the ADP-ribosylating S1 subunit.

5.5 Botulinum C2 Toxin

Receptor-bound component II of botulinum C2 toxin is apparently endocytosed, since it disappears from the cell surface during incubation at 37 °C (SIMPSON 1989). SIMPSON (1989) also found that weak bases such as ammonia and methylamine protected cells against C2 toxin. This was interpreted as an effect due to inhibition of receptor-mediated endocytosis. However, there is currently no evidence that weak bases generally block endocytosis, and one should therefore also consider other reasons why weak bases protect against C2 toxin. One possibility could be that a low intravesicular pH may be required for either a membrane translocation step or a processing event. The oligomeric form of trypsinized component II possesses hemolytic properties (OHISHI 1987). This could reflect insertion into the plasma membrane.

6 Conclusions

It can be concluded that, despite their diversity in size, subunit composition, cell specificity, and substrates, the ADP-ribosylating toxins appear to share a similar multistep mechanism in which (1) the toxin binds to a receptor on the membrane of a target cell, (2) the catalytic domain is translocated into, or at least comes into contact with, the cytoplasm, and (3) the catalytic domain is then able to modify the target substrate.

One of the reasons why cytotoxic ADP-ribosylating proteins have received much attention in later years is their use in preparation of immunotoxins and other chimeras. There is now reason to believe that such molecules may be of great importance in targeted cell killing in cancer and other diseases. However, to be therapeutically useful, chimeras must be specifically targeted, and this will in most cases involve manipulation of the toxin in order to eliminate binding to toxin receptors as such. It will therefore be an important task to pursue the characterization of the binding and translocation mechanisms in as much detail as possible. In particular, it will be crucial to elucidate which parts of the molecules are essential for biological activity, and which parts can be dispensed of without losing activity.

References

Aktories K, Wegner A (1989) ADP-ribosylation of actin by clostridial toxins. J Cell Biol 109: 1385–1387

Aktories K, Barmann M, Ohishi I, Tsuyama S, Jakobs KH, Habermann E (1986) Botulinum C2 toxin ADP-ribosylates actin. Nature 322: 390–392

Allured VS, Collier RJ, Carroll SF, Mckay DB (1986) Structure of exotoxin A of *Pseudomonas aeruginosa* at 3.0-Ångstrom resolution. Proc Natl Acad Sci USA 83: 1320–1324

Arai H, Sato Y (1976) Separation and characterization of two distinct hemagglutinins contained in purified leukosis-promoting factor from *Bordetella pertussis*. Biochim Biophys Acta 444: 765–782

Armstrong GD, Howard LA, Peppler MS (1988) Use of glycosyltransferases to restore pertussis toxin receptor activity to asialogalactofetuin. J Biol Chem 263: 8677–8684

Bennett V, Cuatrecasas P (1975) Mechanism of activation of adenylate cyclase by *Vibrio cholerae* enterotoxin. J Membr Biol 222: 29–52

Blewitt MG, Zhao J-M, McKeever B, Sarma R, London E (1984) fluorescence characterization of the low pH-induced change in diphtheria toxin conformation: effect of salt. Biochem Biophys Res Commun 120: 286–290

Blewitt MG, Chung LA, London E (1985a) Effect of pH on the conformation of diphtheria toxin and its implications for membrane penetration. Biochemistry 24: 5458–5464

Blewitt MG, Chung LA, London E (1985b) Interaction of diphtheria toxin with model membranes. Biochemistry 24: 5458–5464

Boquet P, Pappenheimer AM Jr (1976) Interaction of diptheria toxin with mammalian cell membranes. J Biol Chem 251: 5770–5778

Brennan MJ, David JL, Kenimer JG, Manclark CR (1988) Lectin-like binding of pertussis toxin to a 165-kilodalton Chinese hamster ovary cell glycoprotein. J Biol Chem 263: 4895–4899

Cabiaux V, Brasseur R, Wattiez R, Falmagne P, Ruysschaert J-M, Goormaghtigh E (1989) Secondary structure of diphtheria toxin and its fragments interacting with acidic liposomes studied by polarized infrared spectroscopy. J Biol Chem 264: 4928–4938

Carroll SF, Collier RJ (1988) Amino acid sequence homology between the enzymic domains of diphtheria toxin and *Pseudomonas aeruginosa* exotoxin A. Mol Microbiol 4: 527–535

Cassel D, Pfeuffer T (1978) Mechanism of cholera toxin action: covalent modification of the guanyl nucleotide-binding protein of the adenylate cyclase system. Proc Natl Acad Sci USA 75: 2669–2673

Chaudhary VK, Jinno Y, FitzGerald D, Pastan I (1990) *Pseudomonas* exotoxin contains a specific sequence at the carboxyl terminus that is required for cytotoxicity. Proc Natl Acad Sci USA 87: 308–312

Chaudry GJ, Wilson RB, Draper RK, Clowes RC (1989) A dipeptide insertion in domain I of exotoxin A that impairs receptor binding. J Biol Chem 264: 15151–15156

Cieplak W, Gaudin HM, Eidels L (1987) Diphtheria toxin receptor. Identification of specific diphtheria toxin-binding proteins on the surface of Vero and BS-C-1 cells. J Biol Chem 262: 13246–13253

Collier RJ, Westbrook EM, McKay DB, Eisenberg D (1982) X-ray grade crystals of diphtheria toxin. J Biol Chem 257: 5283–5285

Cuatrecasas P (1977) Interaction of *Vibrio cholerae* enterotoxin with cell membranes. Biochemistry 12: 3547–3558

Dallas WS, Falkow S (1980) Amino acid sequence homology between cholera toxin and *Escherichia coli* heat-labile toxin. Nature 288: 499–501

De Wolf MJS, Fridkin M, Kohn LD (1981) Tryptophan residues of cholera toxin and its A and B protomers. Intrinsic fluorescence and solute quenching upon interacting with the ganglioside GM_1, oligo-GM_1, or dansylated oligo-GM_1. J Biol Chem 256: 5489–5496

Donovan JJ, Simon MI, Draper RK, Montal M (1981) Diphtheria toxin forms transmembrane channels in planar lipid bilayers. Proc Natl Acad Sci USA 78: 172–176

Donovan JJ, Simon MI, Montal M (1985) Requirements for the translocation of diphtheria toxin fragment A across lipid membranes. J Biol Chem 260: 8817–8823

Draper RK, Simon MI (1980) The entry of diphtheria toxin into the mammalian cell cytoplasm: evidence for lysosomal involvement. J Cell Biol 87: 849–854

Drazin R, Kandel J, Collier RJ (1971) Structure and activity of diphtheria toxin. II. Attack by trypsin at a specific site within the intact toxin molecule. J Biol Chem 246: 1504–1510

Duffy LK, Lai CY (1979) Involvement of arginine residues in the binding of cholera toxin subunit B. Biochem Biophys Res Commun 91: 1005–1010

Dumont ME, Richards FM (1988) The pH-dependent conformational change of diphtheria toxin. J Biol Chem 263: 2087–2097

Dwyer JD, Bloomfield VA (1982) Subunit arrangement of cholera toxin in solution and bound to receptor-containing model membranes. Biochemistry 21: 3227–3231

Eidels L, Proia RL, Hart DA (1983) Membrane receptors for bacterial toxins. Microbiol Rev 47: 596–620

Eisenberg D, Schwarz E, Komaromy M, Wall R (1984) Analysis of membrane and surface protein sequences with the hydrophobic moment plot. J Mol Biol 179: 125–142

Farahbakhsh ZT, Baldwin RL, Wisnieski BJ (1986) *Pseudomonas* exotoxin A. Membrane binding, insertion, and traversal. J Biol Chem 261: 11404–11408

Farahbakhsh ZT, Baldwin RL, Wisnieski BJ (1987) Effect of low pH on the conformation of *Pseudomonas* exotoxin A. J Biol Chem 262: 2256–2261

Farfel Z, Kaslow HR, Bourne HR (1979) A regulatory component of adenylate cyclase is located on the inner surface of human erythrocyte membranes. Biochem Biophys Res Commun 90: 1237–1241

Finkelstein RA (1973) Cholera. Crit Rev Microbiol 2: 553–623

Finkelstein RA, Burks MF, Zupan A, Dallas WS, Jacob CO, Ludwig DS (1987) Antigenic determinants of the cholera/coli family of enterotoxins. Rev Infect Dis 9: S490–S502

Fishman PH (1980) Mechanism of action of cholera toxin: studies on the lag period. J Membr Biol 54: 61–72

FitzGerald D, Morris RE, Saelinger CB (1980) Receptor-mediated internalization of *Pseudomonas* toxin by mouse fibroblasts. Cell 21: 867–873

Fukuta S, Magnani JL, Twiddy EM, Holmes RK, Ginsburg V (1988) Comparison of the carbohydrate-binding specificities of cholera toxin and *Escherichia coli* heat-labile enterotoxins LTh-I, LT-IIa, and LT-IIb. Infect Immun 56: 1748–1753

Geary S, Marchlewics BA, Finkelstein RA (1982) Comparisons of heat-labile enterotoxins from porcine and human strains of *Escherichia coli*. Infect Immun 36: 215–220

Gill DM (1976a) The arrangement of subunits in cholera toxin. Biochemistry 15: 1242–1248

Gill DM (1976b) Multiple roles of erythrocyte supernatant in the activation of adenylate cyclase by *Vibrio cholerae* toxin in vitro. J Infect Dis 133: S55–S63

Gill DM (1977) Mechanism of action of cholera toxin. Adv Cyclic Nucleotide Res 8: 85–118

Gill DM, King CA (1975) The mechanism of action of cholera toxin in pigeon erythrocyte lysates. J Biol Chem 250: 6424–6432

Gill DM, Clements JD, Robertson DC, Finkelstein RA (1981) Subunit number and arrangement in *Escherichia coli* heat-labile enterotoxin. Infect Immun 33: 677–682

Gill DM, Meren R (1978) ADP-ribosylation of membrane proteins catalyzed by cholera toxin: basis of the activation of adenylate cyclase. Proc Natl Acad Sci USA 75: 3050–3054

Gray BL, Smith DH, Baldridge JS, Harkins RN, Vasil ML, Chen EY, Heyneker HL (1984) Cloning, nucleotide sequence, and expression in *Escherichia coli* of the exotoxin A structural gene of *Pseudomonas aeruginosa*. Proc Natl Acad Sci USA 81: 2645–2649

Greenfield L, Bjorn MJ, Horn G, Fong D, Buck GA, Collier RJ, Kaplan DA (1983) Nucleotide sequence of the structural gene for diphtheria toxin carried by corynebacteriophage beta. Proc Natl Acad Sci USA 80: 6853–6857

Griffiths SI, Finkelstein RA, Critchley DR (1986) Characterization of the receptor for cholera toxin and *Escherichia coli* heat-labile toxin in rabbit intestinal brush borders. Biochem J 238: 313–322

Guidi-Rontani C, Collier RJ (1987) Exotoxin A of *Pseudomonas aeruginosa*: evidence that domain I functions in receptor binding. Mol Microbiol 1: 67–72

Holmgren J (1973) Tissue receptor for cholera exotoxin: postulated structure from studies with GM_1 ganglioside and related glycolipids. Infect Immun 8: 208–214

Holmgren J (1981) Actions of cholera toxin and the prevention and treatment of cholera. Nature 292: 413–417

Holmgren J, Fredman P, Lindblad M, Svennerholm A-M, Svennerholm L (1982) Rabbit intestinal glycoprotein receptor for *Escherichia coli* heat-labile enterotoxin lacking affinity for cholera toxin. Infect Immun 38: 424–433

Holmgren J, Lindblad M, Fredman P, Svennerholm L, Myrvold H (1985) Comparison of receptors for cholera and *Escherichia coli* enterotoxins in human intestine. Gastroenterology 89: 27–35

Honda T, Tsuji T, Takeda Y, Miwatani T (1981) Immunological nonidentity of heat-labile enterotoxins from human and porcine enterotoxigenic *Escherichia coli*. Infect Immun 34: 337–340

Honjo T, Nishizuka Y, HAyaishi O, Kato I (1968) Diphtheria toxin-dependent adenosine diphosphate ribosylation of aminoacyl transferase II and inhibition of protein synthesis. J Biol Chem 243: 3553–3555

Hu VW, Holmes RK (1984) Evidence for direct insertion of fragments A and B of diphtheria toxin into model membranes J Biol Chem 259: 12226–12233

Hudson TH, Scharff J, Kimak MAG, Neville DM Jr (1988) Energy requirements for diphtheria toxin translocation are coupled to the maintenance of a plasma membrane potential and a proton gradient. J Biol Chem 263: 4773–4781

Hwang J, Fitzgerald DJ, Adhya S, Pastan I (1987) Functional domains of *Pseudomonas* exotoxin identified by deletion analysis of the gene expressed in *E. coli.* Cell 48: 129–136

Idziorek T, FitzGerald D, Pastan I (1990) Low pH-induced changes in *Pseudomonas* exotoxin and its domains: increased binding of triton X-114. Infect Immun 58: 1415–1420

Iglewski BH, Sadoff JC (1979) Toxin inhibitors of protein synthesis: production, purification, and assay of *Pseudomonas aeruginosa* toxin A. Methods Enzymol 60: 780–793

Iida T, Tsuji T, Honda T, Miwatani T, Wakabayashi S, Wada K, Matsubara H (1989) A single amino acid substitution in B subunit of *Escherichia coli* enterotoxin affects its oligomer formation. J Biol Chem 264: 14065–14070

Irons LI, MacLennan AP (1979) Isolation of the lymphocytosis promoting factor-haemagglutinin of *Bordetella pertussis* by affinity chromatography. Biochim Biophys Acta 580: 175–185

Ittelson TR, Gill DM (1973) Diphtheria toxin: specific competition for receptors. Nature 242: 330–331

Jacob CO, Sela M, Arnon R (1983) Antibodies against synthetic peptides of the B subunit of cholera toxin: crossreaction and neutralization of the toxin. Proc Natl Acad Sci USA 80: 7611–7615

Jacob CO, Pines M, Arnon R (1984) Neutralization of heat-labile toxin of *E-coli* by antibodies to synthetic peptides derived from the B subunit of cholera toxin. EMBO J 3: 2889–2893

Janicot M, Fouque F, Des Buquois B (1991) Activation of rat liver adenylate cyclase by cholera toxin requires toxin internalization and processing in endosomes. J Biol Chem 266: 12858–12865

Jiang JX, London E (1990) Involvement of denaturation-like changes in *Pseudomonas* exotoxin A hydrophobicity and membrane penetration determined by characterization pH and thermal transitions. J Biol Chem 265: 8636–8641

Jinno Y, Chaudhary VK, Kondo T, Adhya S, FitzGerald DJ, Pastan I (1988) Mutational analysis of domain I of *Pseudomonas* exotoxin. Mutations in domain I of *Pseudomonas* exotoxin which reduce cell binding and animal toxicity. J Biol Chem 263:13203–13207

Joseph KC, Kim Su, Stieber A, Gonatas NK (1978) Endocytosis of cholera toxin into neuronal GERL. Proc Natl Acad Sci USA 75: 2815–2819

Kagan B, Finkelstein A, Colombini M (1981) Diphtheria toxin fragment forms large pores in phospholipid bilayer membranes. Proc Natl Acad Sci USA 78: 4950–4954

Kassis S, Hagmann J, Fishman PH, Chang PP, Moss J (1982) Mechanism of action of cholera toxin on intact cells. Generation of A_1 peptide and activation of adenylate cyclase. J Biol Chem 257: 12148–12152

Kim K, Groman NB (1965) In vitro inhibition of diphtheria toxin action by ammonium salts and amines. J Bacteriol 90: 1552–1556

Kimberg DV, Field M, Johnson J, Henderson A, Gershon E (1971) Stimulation of intestinal mucosal adenyl cyclase by cholera enterotoxin and prostaglandins. Clin Invest 50: 1218–1231

Kohno K, Hayes H, Mekada E, Uchida T (1987) Mutant with diphtheria toxin receptor and acidification function but defective in entry of toxin. Exp Cell Res 172: 54–64

Kurosky A, Markel De, Peterson JW (1977a) Covalent structure of the B chain of cholera enterotoxin. J Biol Chem 252: 7257–7264

Kursoky A, Markel DE, Peterson JW, Fitch WM (1977b) Primary structure of cholera toxin B-chain: a glycoprotein hormone analog? Science 195: 299–301

Lai C-Y (1977) Determination of the primary structure of cholera toxin B subunit. J Biol Chem 252: 7249–7256

Lai C-Y (1980) The chemistry and biology of cholera toxin. CRC Crit Rev Biochem 9: 171–206

Lambotte P, Falmagne P, Capiau C, Zanen J, Ruysschaert JM, Dirkx J (1980) Primary structure of diphtheria toxin fragment B: structural similarities with lipid-binding domains. J Cell Biol 87: 837–840

Leong J, Vinal AC, Dallas WS (1985) Nucleotide sequences comparison between heat-labile toxin B-subunit cistrons from *Escherichia coli* of human and porcine origin. Infect Immun 48: 73–77

Leppla SH, Dorland RB, Middlebrook JL (1980) Inhibition of diphtheria toxin degradation and cytotoxic action by chloroquine. J Biol Chem 255: 2247–2250

Locht C, Keith JM (1986) Pertussis toxin gene: nucleotide sequence and genetic organization. Science 232: 1258–1264

Lockman H, Kaper JB (1983) Nucleotide sequence analysis of the A2 and B subunits of *Vibrio cholerae* enterotoxin. J Biol Chem 258: 13722–13726

Ludwig DS, Holmes RK, Schoolnik GK (1985) Chemical and immunochemical studies on the receptor binding domain of cholera toxin B subunit. J Biol Chem 260: 12528–12534

Madshus IH, Collier RJ (1989) Effects of eliminating a disulfide bridge within domain II of *Pseudomonas aeruginosa* exotoxin A. Infect Immun 57: 1873–1878

Manhart MD, Morris RE, Bonventre PF, Leppla S, Saelinger CB (1984) Evidence for *Pseudomonas* exotoxin A receptors on plasma membrane of toxin-sensitive LM fibroblasts. Infect Immun 45: 596–603

Marnell MH, Stookey M, Draper RK (1982) Monensin blocks the transport of diphtheria toxin to the cell cytoplasm. J Cell Biol 93: 57–62

Marnell MH, Mathis LS, Stookey M, Shia SP, Stone DK, Draper RK (1984a) A chinese hamster ovary cell mutant with heat-sensitive conditional-lethal defect in vacuolar function. J Cell Biol 99: 1907–1916

Marnell MH, Shia SP, Stookey M, Draper RK (1984b) Evidence for penetration of diphtheria toxin to the cytosol through a prelysosomal membrane. Infect Immun 44: 145–150

Maulik PR, Reed RA, Shipley GG (1988) Crystallization and preliminary X-ray diffraction study of cholera toxin B-subunit. J Biol Chem 263: 9499–9501

McGill S, Stenmark H, Sandvig K, Olsnes S (1989) Membrane interactions of diphtheria toxin analyzed using in vitro translated mutants. EMBO J 8: 2843–2848

Mekada E, Uchida T (1985) Binding properties of diphtheria toxin to cells are altered by mutation in the fragment A domain. J Biol Chem 260: 12148–12153

Mekada E, Uchida T, Okada Y (1981) Methylamine stimulates the action of ricin toxin but inhibits that of diphtheria toxin. J Biol Chem 256: 1225–1228

Mekada E, Okada Y, Uchida T (1988) Identification of diphtheria toxin receptor and a nonproteinous diphtheria toxin-binding molecule in Vero cell membrane. J Cell Biol 107: 511–519

Mekalanos JJ, Collier RJ, Romig WR (1979) Enzymic activity of cholera toxin. II. Relationships to proteolytic processing, disulfide bond reduction, and subunit composition. J Biol Chem 254: 5855–5861

Mekalanos JJ, Swartz DJ, Pearson GDN, Harford N, Groyne F, de Wilde M (1983) Cholera toxin genes: nucleotide sequence, deletion analysis and vaccine development. Nature 306: 551–557

Merion M, Schlesinger P, Brooks RM, Moehring JM, Moehring TJ, Sly WS (1983) Defective acidification of endosomes in Chinese hamster ovary cell mutants "cross-resistant" to toxins and Viruses. Proc Natl Acad Sci USA 80: 5315–5319

Middlebrook JL, Doorland RB (1984) Bacterial toxins: cellular mechanisms of action. Microbiol Rev 48: 199–221

Middlebrook JL, Doorland RB, Leppla SH (1978) Association of diphtheria toxin with Vero cells: demonstration of a receptor. J Biol Chem 253: 7325–7330

Moehring, TJ, Crispell JB (1974) Enzyme treatment of KB cells: the altered effect of diphtheria toxin. Biochem Biophys Res Commun 60: 1446–1452

Montecucco C, Schiavo G, Tomasi M (1985) pH-dependence of the phospholipid interaction of diphtheria toxin fragments. Biochem J 231: 123–128

Montecucoo C, Tomasi M, Schiavo G, Rappuoli R (1986) Hydrophobic photolabelling of pertussis toxin subunits interacting with lipids. FEBS Lett 194: 301–304

Montesano R, Roth J, Robert A, Orci L (1982) Non-coated membrane invaginations are involved in binding and internalization of cholera and tetanus toxins. Nature 296: 651–653

Morris RE, Saelinger CB (1986) Reduced temperature alters *Pseudomonas* exotoxin A entry into the mouse LM cell. Infect Immun 52: 445–453

Morris RE, Manhart MD, Saelinger CB (1983) Receptor-mediated entry of *Pseudomonas* toxin: methylamine blocks clustering step. Infect Immun 40: 806–811

Morris RE, Gerstein AS, Bonventre PF, Saelinger CB (1985) Receptor-mediated entry of diphtheria toxin into monkey kidney (Vero) cells: electron microscopic evaluation. Infect Immun 50: 721 727

Moskaug JØ, Sandvig K, Olsnes S (1987) Cell-mediated reduction of the interfragment disulfide in nicked diphtheria toxin. A new system to study toxin entry at low pH. J Biol Chem 262: 10339–10345

Moskaug JØ, Sandvig K, Olsnes S (1988) Low pH-induced release of diphtheria toxin A-fragment in Vero cells. Biochemical evidence for transfer to the cytosol. J Biol Chem 263: 2518–2525

Moskaug JØ, Stenmark H, Olsnes S (1991) Insertion of diphtheria toxin B-fragment into the plasma membrane at low pH. Characterization and topology of inserted regions. J Biol Chem 266: 2652–2659

Moss J, Vaughan M (1977) Mechanism of action of choleragen. Evidence for ADP-ribosyltransferase activity with arginine as an acceptor. J Biol Chem 252: 2455–2457

Moss J, Vaughan M (1988) ADP-ribosylation of guanyl nucleotide-binding regulatory proteins by bacterial toxins. Adv Enzymol 61: 303–379

Moss J, Stanley SJ, Morin JE, Dixon JE (1980) Activation of choleragen by thiol: protein disulfide oxidoreductase. J Biol Chem 255: 11085–11087

Moya M, Dautry-Varsat A, Goud B, Louvard D, Boquet P (1985) Inhibition of coated pit formation in Hep2 cells blocks the cytotoxicity of diphtheria toxin but not that of ricin toxin. J Cell Biol 101: 548–559

Moynihan MR, Pappenheimer AM Jr (1991) Kinetics of adenosine-diphosphorylation of elongation factor 2 in cells exposed to diphtheria toxin. Infect Immun 32: 575–582

Mullin BR, Aloj SM, Fishman PH, Lee G, Kohn LD (1976) Cholera toxin interactions with thyrotropin receptors on thyroid plasma membranes. Proc Natl Acad Sci USA 73: 1679–1683

Munro S, Pelham RB (1987) A C-terminal signal prevents secretion of luminal ER proteins. Cell 48: 899–907

Murphy JR, Bishai W, Borowski M, Miyanohara A, Boyd J, Nagle S (1986) Genetic construction, expression, and melanoma-selective cytotoxity of a diphtheria toxin-related a-melanocyte-stimulating hormone fusion protein. Proc Natl Acad Sci USA 83: 8258–8262

Nicosia A, Perugini M, Franzini C, Casagli MC, Borri MG, Antoni G, Almoni M, Neri P, Ratti G, Rappuoli R (1986) Cloning and sequencing of the pertussis toxin genes: Operon structure and gene duplication. Proc Natl Acad Sci USA 83: 4631–4635

Ohishi I (1987) Activation of botulinum C2 toxin by trypsin. Infect Immun 55: 1461–1465

Ohishi I, Miyake M (1985) Binding of the two components of C2 toxin to epithelial cells and brush borders of mouse intestine. Infect Immun 48: 769–775

Ohishi I, Iwasaki M, Sakaguchi G (1980) Purification and characterization of two components of botulinum C2 toxin. Infect Immun 30: 668–673

O'Keefe DO, Collier RJ (1989) Cloned diphtheria toxin within the periplasm of *Escherichia coli* causes lethal membrane damage at low pH. Proc Natl Acad Sci USA 86: 343–346

Olsnes S, Carvajal E, Sundan A, Sandvig K (1985) Evidence that membrane phospholipids and protein are required for binding of diphtheria toxin in Vero cells. Biochim Biophys Acta 846: 334–341

Olsnes S, Carvajal E, Sandvig K (1986) Interactions between diphtheria toxin entry and anion transport in Vero cells. III. Effect on toxin binding and anion transport of tumor-promoting phorbol esters, vanadate, fluoride, and salicylate. J Biol Chem 261: 1562–1569

Papini E, Schiavo G, Tomasi M, Colombatti M, Rappuoli R, Montecucco C (1987) Lipid interactions of diphtheria toxin and mutants with altered fragment B. II. Hydrophobic photolabelling and cell intoxication. Eur J Biochem 169: 637–644

Papini E, Sandona D, Rappuoli R, Montecucco C (1988) On the membrane translocation of diphtheria toxin: at low pH the toxin induces ion channels on cells. EMBO J 7(11): 3353–3359

Patzer EJ, Wagner RR, Dubovi EJ (1979) Viral membranes: model systems for studying biological membranes. CRC Crit Rev Biochem 8: 165–217

Pirker R, FitzGerald DJP, Hamilton TC, Ozols RF, Willingham MC, Pastan I (1985) Anti-transferrin receptor antibody linked to *Pseudomonas* exotoxin as a model immunotoxin in human ovarian carcinoma cell lines. Cancer Res 45: 751–757

Proia RL, Hart DA, Holmes RK, Holmes KV, Eidels L (1979) Immunoprecipitation and partial characterization of diphtheria toxin-binding glycoproteins from surface of guinea pig cells. Proc natl Acad Sci USA 76: 685–689

Ratti G, Rappuoli R, Giannini G (1983) The complete sequence of the gene for diphtheria toxin in the corynephage omega (tox+) genome. Nucleic Acids Res 11: 6589–6595

Ribi Ho, Ludwig DS, Mercer KL, Schoolnik GK, Kornberg RD (1988) Three-dimensional structure of cholera toxin penetrating a lipid membrane. Science 239: 1272–1276

Robbins AR, Peng SS, Marshall JL (1983) Mutant Chinese hamster ovary cells pleiotropically defective in receptor-mediated endocytosis. J Cell Biol 96: 1064–1071

Robbins AR, Oliver C, Bateman JL, Krag SS, Galloway CJ, Mellman I (1984) A single mutation in Chinese hamster ovary cells impairs both golgi and endosomal functions. J Cell Biol 99: 1296–1308

Robles CP, Hart DA, Eidels L (1982) Diphtheria toxin-binding cell surface glycoproteins. Fed Proc 41: 1392

Robles CP, Hart DA, Eidels L (1983) Diphtheria toxin-binding glycoproteins on the surface of cells in culture. Fed Proc 42: 1809

Roff CF, Fuchs R, Mellman I, Robbins AR (1986) Chinese hamster ovary cell mutants with temperature-sensitive defects in endocytosis. I. Loss of function on shifting to the nonpermissive temperature. J Cell Biol 103: 2283–2297

Rolf JM, Gaudin HM, Tirrell SM, MacDonald AB, Eidels L (1989) Anti-idiotypic antibodies that protect cells against the action of diphtheria toxin. Proc Natl Acad Sci USA 86: 2036–2039

Rolf JM, Gaudin HM, Eidels L (1990) Localization of the diphtheria toxin receptor-binding domain to the carboxyl-terminal $M_r \sim 6000$ region of the toxin. J Biol Chem 265: 7331–7337

Sandvig K, Moskaug JØ (1987) *Pseuodomonas* toxin binds Triton X-114 at low pH. Biochem J 245: 899–901

Sandvig K, Olsnes S (1980) Diphtheria toxin entry into cells is facilitated by low pH. J Cell Biol 87: 828–832

Sandvig K, Olsnes S (1981) Rapid entry of nicked diphtheria toxin into cells at low pH. Characterization of the entry process and effect of low pH on the toxin molecule. J Biol Chem 256: 9068–9076

Sandvig K, Olsnes S (1984) Anion requirements and effect of anion transport inhibitors on the response of Vero cells to diphtheria toxin and modeccin. J Cell Physiol 119: 7–14

Sandvig K, Olsnes S, (1986) Interactions between diphtheria toxin entry and anion transport in Vero cells. IV. Evidence that entry of diphtheria toxin is dependent on efficient anion transport. J Biol Chem 261: 1570–1575

Sandvig K, Olsnes S (1988) Diphtheria toxin-induced channels in Vero cells selective for monovalent cations. J Biol Chem 263: 12352–12359

Sandvig K, Olsnes S (1991) Membrane translocation of diphtheria toxin. In: Alouf JE, Freer JH (eds) Sourcebook of bacterial protein toxins. Academic Press Limited, London, UK, pp 57–73

Sandvig K, Sundan A, Olsnes S (1984) Evidence that diphtheria toxin and modeccin enter the cytosol from different vesicular compartments. J Cell Biol 98: 963–970

Sandvig K, Tønnessen TI, Sand O, Olsnes S (1986) Requirement of a transmembrane pH gradient for the entry of diphtheria toxin into cells at low pH. J Biol Chem 261: 11639–11644

Schaefer EM, Moehring JM, Moehring TJ (1988) Binding of diphtheria toxin to CHO-KI and Vero cells is dependent on cell density. J Cell Physiol 135: 407–415

Sekura RD, Fish F, Manclark CR, Meade B, Zhang Y (1983) Pertussis toxin. Affinity purification of a new ADP-ribosyltransferase. J Biol Chem 258: 14647–14651

Siegall CB, Chaudhary VK, FitzGerald DJ, Pastan I (1989) Functional analysis of domains II, Ib, and III of *Pseudomonas* exotoxin. J Biol Chem 264: 14256–14261

Sigler PB, Druyan ME, Kiefer HC, Finkelstein RA (1977) Cholera toxin crystals suitable for X-ray diffraction. Science 197: 1277–1279

Simpson LI (1989) The binary toxin produced by *Clostridium botulinum* enters cells by receptor-mediated endocytosis to exert its pharmacologic effects. J Pharmacol Exp Ther 251: 1223–1228

Sixma TK, Pronk SE, Kalk KH, Wartna ES, Van Zanten BAM, Witholt B, Hol WGJ (1991) Crystal structure of cholera toxin related heat labile enterotoxin from E. coli. Nature 351: 371–377

Stenmark H, McGill S, Olsnes S, Sandvig K (1989) Plasma membrane permeabilization by deletion mutants of diphtheria toxin. EMBO J 8: 2849–2853

Sundan A, Sandvig K, Olsnes S (1984) Calmodulin antagonists sensitize cells to *Pseudomonas* toxin. J Cell Physiol 119: 15–22

Svennerholm A-M, Holmgren J (1978) Identification of *Escherichia coli* heat-labile enterotoxin by means of a ganglioside immunosorbent assay (GM_1-ELISA) procedure. Curr Microbiol 1: 19–23

Takao T, Watanabe H, Shimonishi Y (1985) Facile identification of protein sequences by mass spectrometry. B subunit of *Vibrio cholerae* classical biotype Inaba 569 B toxin. Eur J Biochem 146: 503–508

Tamura M, Nogimori K, Yajima M, Ito K, Katada T, Ui M, Ishii S (1982) Subunit structure of islet-activating protein, pertussis toxin, in conformity with the A-B model. Biochemistry 21: 5516–5522

Thompson MR, Forristal J, Kauffmann P, Madden T, Kozak K, Morris R, Saelinger CB (1991) Isolation and characterization of *Pseudomonas aeruginosa* exotoxin A binding glycoprotein from mouse LM cells. J Biol Chem 266: 2390–2396

Tomasi M, Montecucco C (1981) Lipid insertion of cholera toxin after binding to GM_1-containing lipsosomes. J Biol Chem 256: 11177–11181

Tomasi M, Battistini A, Ausiello C, Roda LG, d'Angolo GD (1978) The role of environmental parameters on the stability of cholera toxin functional regions. FEBS Lett 94: 253–256

Tosteson MT, Tosteson DC (1978) Bilayers containing gangliosides develop channels when exposed to cholera toxin. Nature 275: 142–144

Tsuji T, Honda T, Miwatani T, Wakabayashi S, Matsubara H (1984) The amino acid sequence of the B-subunit: of porcine enterotoxigenic *Escherichia coli* enterotoxin- analysis and comparison with literature data. FEMS Microbiol Lett 25: 243–246

Tsuji T, Honda T, Miwatani T, Wakabayashi S, Matsubara H (1985) Analysis of receptor-binding site in *Escherichia coli* enterotoxin. J Biol Chem 260: 8552–8558

Tsuji T, Iida T, Honda T, Miwatani T, Nagahama M, Sakurai J, Wada K, Matsubara H (1987) A unique amino acid sequence of the B subunit of a heat-labile enterotoxin isolated from a human enterotoxigenic *Escherichia coli.* Microb Pathog 2: 381–390

Uchida T, Pappenheimer AM Jr, Harper AA (1972) Reconstitution of diphtheria toxin from two nontoxic cross-reacting molecules. Science 175: 901–903

Uchida T, Pappenheimer AM Jr, Greany R (1973) Diphtheria toxin and related proteins. I. Isolation and properties of mutant proteins serologically related to diphtheria toxin. J Biol Chem 248: 3838–3844

Van Heynigen WE, Carpenter CCJ, Pierce NF, Greenough WB III (1971) Deactivation of cholera toxin by ganglioside. J Infect Dis 124: 415–418

Van Ness BG, Howard JB, Bodley JW (1980) ADP-ribosylation of elongation factor 2 by diphtheria toxin. NMR spectra and proposed structures of ribosyl-diphthamide and its hydrolysis products. J Biol Chem 255: 10710–10716

Wick MJ, Hammond AN, Iglewski BH (1990) MIcroReview. Analysis of the structure-function relationship of *Pseudomonas aeruginosa* exotoxin A. Mol Microbiol 4: 527–535

Wisnieski BJ, Bramhall JS (1981) Photolabelling of cholera toxin subunits during membrane penetration. Nature 289: 319–321

Yamamoto T, Yokota T (1983) Sequence of heat-labile enterotoxin of *Escherichia coli* pathogenic for humans. J Bacteriol 155: 728–733

Yamamoto T, Gojobori T, Yokota T (1987) Evolutionary origin of pathogenic determinants in enterotoxigenic *Escherichia coli* and *Vibrio cholerae* 01. J Bacteriol 169: 1352–1357

Zhao J-M, London E (1986) Similarity of the conformation of diphtheria toxin at high temperature to that in the membrane-penetrating low-pH state. Proc Natl Acad Sci USA 83: 2002–2006

Zhao J-M, London E (1988) Conformation and model membrane interactions of diphtheria toxin, fragment A. J Biol Chem 263: 15369–15377

Diphtheria Toxin and *Pseudomonas aeruginosa* Exotoxin A: Active-Site Structure and Enzymic Mechanism

B. A. WILSON and R. J. COLLIER

1 Introduction

Diphtheria toxin (DT), secreted by lysogenic strains of *Corynebacterium diphtheriae* carrying the phage-encoded DT gene, was the first ADP-ribosylating toxin for which the molecular mechanism of action was elucidated (COLLIER 1975; PAPPENHEIMER 1977), and for many years DT has served as an important model system for studying the pathogenesis of bacterial exotoxins (COLLIER 1982; JACOBSON and JACOBSON 1989; MOSS and VAUGHAN 1990). DT and the closely related exotoxin A from *Pseudomonas aeruginosa* (ETA) both catalyze the ADP-ribosylation of a post-translationally modified histidine (diphthamide) on elongation factor 2 (EF-2) (HONJO et al. 1968, 1969; GILL et al. 1969; IGLEWSKI and KABAT 1975; IGLEWSKI et al. 1977). EF-2 is a GTP-binding protein involved in protein biosynthesis by eukaryotic cells. ADP-ribosylated EF-2 is no longer able to mediate polypeptide chain elongation, and consequently, toxin-treated cells lose the ability to synthesize protein and ultimately die. Although the catalytic mechanism(s) of the modification reaction and the active sites of these

Department of Microbiology and Molecular Genetics, Harvard Medical School and Shipley Institute of Medicine, 260 Longwood Avenue, Boston, MA 02115, USA

Current Topics in Microbiology and Immunology, Vol. 175

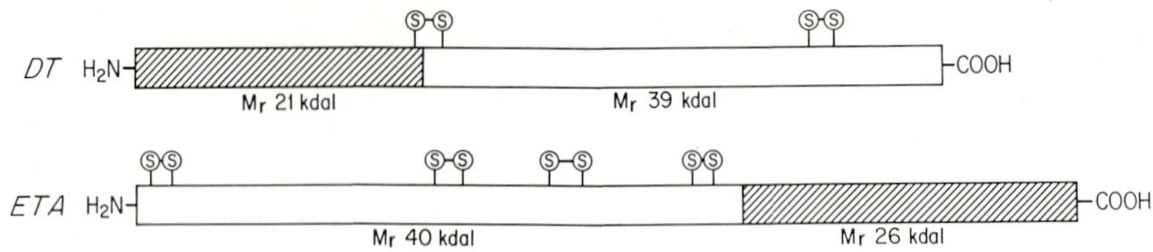

Fig. 1. Schematic representation of DT and ETA, showing the structural differences between the two proteins. The *crosshatched portions* represent the catalytic A moieties; the *remaining portions* represent the B moieties involved in binding and translocation

toxins have not yet been described in detail, recent studies have yielded relevant information. This chapter will focus on some of the more recent studies and what the findings tell us about the structure of the active site and the nature of the reaction catalyzed by these toxins.

2 Structure of DT and ETA Active Sites

For DT and ETA, the receptor-binding, membrane translocation, and enzymatic activity functions are located in separate structural domains within a single, monomeric polypeptide molecule (Fig. 1). Native DT (M_r 58342) and ETA (M_r 66583) are each secreted as proenzymes of 535 and 613 amino acid residues, respectively, which must undergo covalent and/or conformational changes before they can exhibit enzymatic activity. DT activation requires both reduction and partial proteolysis to release the enzymatically active fragment A (GILL and PAPPENHEIMER 1971; COLLIER and KANDEL 1971; DRAZIN et al. 1971), whereas activation of ETA in vitro can be achieved either by disulfide bond reduction in the presence of denaturing agents or by partial proteolytic cleavage (VASIL et al. 1977; CHUNG and COLLIER 1977a; LEPPLA et al. 1978; LORY and COLLIER 1980).

2.1 Structural Differences

DT and ETA show major structural differences (Fig. 1). Their catalytic and receptor-binding domains are located at opposite ends of the molecules, with the catalytic domain being at the amino terminus in DT and at the carboxyl terminus in ETA. The two toxins appear to bind to different target cell surface receptors (MIDDLEBROOK and DORLAND 1977a, b; VASIL and IGLEWSKI 1978; EIDELS et al. 1983). Their amino acid sequences are highly divergent (GREENFIELD et al. 1983; GRAY et al. 1984), and immunologically the two toxins show very little, if any, cross-reactivity (SADOFF et al. 1982). However, despite these differences, there is now considerable evidence that their catalytic domains do indeed share significant sequence homology (CARROLL and COLLIER 1988; GILL 1988; ALLURED et al. 1987; ZHAO and LONDON 1988; DOMENIGHINI et al. 1991), particularly within the active-site cleft, as determined by structure analysis of native ETA, for which there is an X-ray crystal structure available at 3.0-Å resolution (ALLURED et al. 1986). This is consistent with the remarkably similar enzymatic properties of these two toxins. Kinetic constants and inhibitor specificities are similar (COLLIER 1975; KANDEL et al. 1974; CHUNG and COLLIER 1977a, b; COLLIER 1982; LORY et al. 1980; DOUGLAS and COLLIER 1990; WILSON et al. 1990b), with specificity for both protein (EF-2) and NAD substrates being very high ($K_{M(NAD)}$ ca. 9 μ*M* for DT and ca. 35 μ*M* for ETA; $K_{m(EF\text{-}2)}$ ca. 1 μ*M* for both DT and ETA); the stereochemistry of ADP-ribosyl transfer is identical (IGLEWSKI et al. 1977; VAN NESS et al. 1980a, b; OPPENHEIMER and BODLEY 1981); and in the absence of EF-2 substrate, both toxins catalyze the slower reaction of NAD glycohydrolysis (KANDEL et al. 1974; CHUNG and COLLIER 1977a; LORY et al. 1980). The presence of a single, highly specific binding site for NAD, which is responsible for both the ADP-ribosyltransferase and NAD-glycohydrolase activities of the two toxins, was confirmed when an important glutamic acid residue, necessary for catalyzing the ADP-ribosylation of EF-2, was located in each of the toxins' catalytic domains by a unique photoaffinity labeling reaction.

3 Active-Site Studies of DT and ETA

3.1 Identification of a Catalytically Important Glutamic Acid

When complexes of DT fragment A (DTA; 21 kDa) with NAD were irradiated at 254 nm, Glu-148 was specifically and efficiently photolabeled (CARROLL and COLLIER 1984). The photoaddition product formed at position 148 was found to contain the entire nicotinamide moiety of NAD covalently linked, through its C-6, to the decarboxylated γ-methylene carbon of the glutamic acid residue (CARROLL et al. 1985). This structure suggested that the member atoms of the new C—C bond formed in the photoreaction are in close proximity in the DTA-NAD complex that is generated in the initial step of ADP-ribosylation of EF-2. This further suggested that the carboxyl group of Glu-148 might be in contact with the positively charged nitrogen center of NAD and the N-glycosidic bond ruptured during catalysis, implying that Glu-148 might, in fact, participate directly in catalysis. The same photoaffinity labeling technique was subsequently applied to an enzymatically active thermolysin fragment of ETA (ETA-A_{tl}, 27 kDa), resulting in the identification of an analogous active-site glutamic acid residue at position 553 (CARROLL and COLLIER 1987). When Glu-148 of DT was aligned with Glu-553 of ETA (Fig. 2), a local region of amino acid sequence homology was revealed within the proposed active sites of the

```
                                            400        410        420
ETA                                        TGAEFLGDGGDVSFSTRGTQNWTVERLLQAHRQL

DT                                                                 GADDVVDSSK
                                                                           10

    430       440       450          460       470       480       490
ETA  EERGYVFVGYHGTFLEAAQSIVFGGVRARS---QDLDAIWRGFYIAGDPALAYGYAQDQEPDARGRIRNGA
           O *O●OO  * **OO  O  ***O    * O* ●*OO● ***    O O●* O*O   *O  **O*
DT   SFVMENFSSYHGTKPGYVDSIQKGIQKPKSGTQGNYDDDWKGFYSTDNKYDAAGYSVDNENPLSG--KAGG
              20        30        40        50        60        70          80

     500                510       520          530         540       550
ETA  LLRVYVP--------RSSLPGFYRTSLTLAAPEA-AGEV--ERLIGH--PLPLRLDAITGPEEEGGRLETILG
     ***O  O        * * **  ***O*O* *O*  **O  O *O *    * O*      *●*****● O *
DT   VVKVTYPGLTKVLALKVDNAETIKKELGLSLTEPLMEQVGTEEFIKRFGDGASRVVLSLPFAEGSSSVEYINN
              90       100       110       120       130       140       150

     560       570       580       590       600       610
ETA  WPLAERTVVIPSAIPTDPRNVGGDLDPSSIPDKEQAISALPDYASQPGKPPREDLK
     ●  ***** *  *O  **O*  O*
DT   WE-QAKALSVELEINFETRGKRGQDAMYEYMAQACAGNRVRR
           160       170       180       190
```

Fig. 2. Sequence alignment between the catalytic domains of DT and ETA. ○, identical residues; *, conservative substitutions; ●, active-site residues that have been examined by site-directed mutagenesis; *underlined* residues define the loop region that has been examined by substitution and deletion analysis

catalytic domains (CARROLL and COLLIER 1988; GILL 1988; BRANDHUBER et al. 1988; ZHAO and LONDON 1988; DOMENIGHINI et al. 1991). Examination of the X-ray crystallographic structure of native ETA indicated that Glu-553 was indeed located within the presumed active-site cleft of the catalytic domain III of ETA (Fig. 3). A functionally similar and presumably homologous residue in the S-1 subunit of pertussis toxin (PT) has recently been identified (Glu-129) by the same photolabeling reaction (BARBIERI et al. 1989; COCKLE 1989; CIEPLAK et al. 1990).

In both DT and ETA, as well as PT, the putative active-site glutamic acid residues have been subjected to site-directed mutagenesis and biochemical analysis. When aspartic acid or serine was substituted for Glu-148 in the cloned F2 fragment of DT in *Escherichia coli*, the ADP-ribosyltransferase activity of the derived mutant fragment A in crude extracts was found to be less than 1% that of wild-type DTA (TWETEN et al. 1985; BARBIERI and COLLIER 1987). Each mutation produced no alteration in protein stability as measured by protease sensitivity or immunoreactivity, and there was negligible reduction in affinity for NAD. Additionally, the cloned, whole mutant DT, containing the serine substitution at position 148, was found to exhibit an 800-fold decrease in cytotoxicity for cultured BS-C-1 cells (African green monkey kidney cells), a level commensurate with the reduction in ADP-ribosyltransferase activity. The similar substitution of aspartic acid for Glu-553 in ETA (DOUGLAS and COLLIER, 1987, 1990) caused a 3000-fold reduction in ADP-ribosyltransferase activity for the purified ETA-A_{tl}, with a corresponding 400 000-fold decrease in cytotoxicity for mouse L-M cells for whole mutant ETA. Replacement of Glu-553 with cysteine (LUKAC and COLLIER 1988b) or deletion (LUKAC et al. 1988) of the glutamic acid residue resulted in an even greater reduction ($>10^5$-fold) in both enzymic activity and cytotoxicity using crude extracts of mutant toxin. Substitution of Glu-129 in the S-1 subunit of PT with aspartic acid or glycine have likewise been shown to render PT devoid of ADP-ribosylating activity (PIZZA et al. 1988; BARBIERI et al. 1989; CIEPLAK et al. 1990). So, it appears that in these toxins, and perhaps in other ADP-ribosylating toxins as well, there is an active-site glutamic acid residue that is important for catalysis of ADP-ribosylation, since even the most conservative mutations at the active-site glutamic acid have been demonstrated to drastically diminish ADP-ribosylation of EF-2, without significantly affecting substrate binding or protein stability.

In recent work, more detailed kinetic studies have yielded important information on the role of the active-site glutamic acid in catalysis. Additionally, with the aid of the X-ray crystallographic model of ETA and the considerable sequence homology between the active sites of DT and ETA, other potentially important residues in the active-site pocket have been identified, and a systematic analysis of these residues has begun. So far, the results obtained have helped in understanding the structure of the active site and in defining the detailed enzymic mechanism of ADP-ribosylation of EF-2. Current data suggest that the ADP-ribosylation of EF-2 catalyzed by DT and ETA occurs via a direct S_N2 displacement mechanism, involving nucleophilic attack by the nitrogen at position 1 of the imidazole of diphthamide on EF-2, and that the

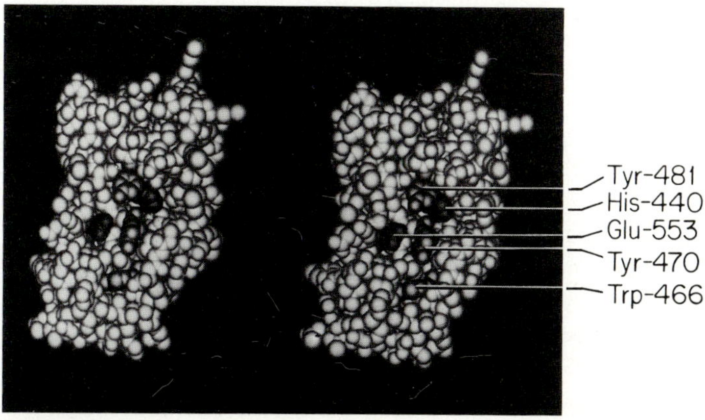

Fig. 3. Stereoview of the active-site cleft of ETA, with Glu-553, Tyr-470, Tyr-481, His-440, and Trp-466 indicated. The model shown was generated from the crystallographic model of ALLURED et al. (1986), with the Promodeler I molecular graphics program (New England BioGraphics. Peacham, VT, USA). Atomic coordinates were provided by David McKay

toxins' active-site glutamic acid carboxyl group is near the disrupted bond and appears to play a crucial role in catalysis of this reaction.

More detailed studies on the catalytic properties of purified mutant forms of DTA have clearly demonstrated the functional importance of this residue for catalysis of ADP-ribosylation. Replacement of Glu-148 with either aspartic acid, glutamine or serine (WILSON et al. 1990b) greatly diminished activity (100- to 300-fold), while producing only minimal changes in K_m or K_d for NAD or K_m for EF-2. The retention of substrate affinities implied that the mutations did not result in major distortions of the overall protein conformation and that the major effects of the mutations were confined to k_{cat}. Even relatively conservative changes, such as withdrawal of the carboxyl group at position 148 by one methylene unit, as in the aspartate mutant, or replacement of the carboxyl group by an uncharged amide, as in the glutamine mutant, were shown to virtually abolish activity. This implied that the precise spatial position and charge of the carboxyl group are crucial for catalysis. Failure of the isosteric glutamine to function effectively in place of glutamic acid further suggested that it is not the hydrogen-bond-forming capability of the carboxyl group, but rather its acidic function, which is important for catalysis. The somewhat greater activity of the aspartic acid mutant over the glutamine mutant supported this proposal.

Surprisingly, these same mutations had virtually no effect on the single substrate NAD-glycohydrolase reaction (WILSON et al. 1990b); only a ten-fold reduction in activity was observed for the serine mutant, and the aspartic acid and glutamine mutants actually exhibited a small, but reproducible increase (ca. 1.7-fold) in NAD-glycohydrolase activity. Since it is unlikely that NAD is bound differently for ADP-ribosylation than for NAD glycohydrolysis, the results suggested that this reaction may proceed by a different mechanism than that of the ADP-ribosylation reaction. Considering the large difference in the observed k_{cat} for these reactions, it was suggested that NAD-glycohydrolase activity may represent a side reaction caused by distortion of the NAD molecule upon binding to DTA, which might facilitate the hydrolytic process. There is no evidence that the weak NAD-glycohydrolase activity has any physiological significance.

The nature of the catalytic function of the glutamic acid has also been studied (WILSON et al. 1990b) by examining the pH dependence of k_{cat} and k_{cat}/K_m of the ADP-ribosylation reaction of DTA for the wild-type protein and the glutamine and serine active-site mutants. Of several conceivable ways in which the carboxyl group might function in catalyzing the ADP-ribosylation of EF-2, initial proposals involved mechanisms in which the carboxyl group served as a general base catalyst. For example, it could function as a base to electrostatically stabilize the quaternary nitrogen center of NAD or a cationic transition-state intermediate, such as an oxycarbonium species, in an S_N1-like mechanism. Alternatively, the carboxylate might serve to deprotonate the incoming diphthamide in an S_N2-type displacement reaction or to maintain important hydrogen-bonding interactions or conformational structure of the active site necessary for catalysis to occur. The inversion of configuration observed at C-1 of ribose in NAD for the ADP-ribosyl transfer reaction (OPPENHEIMER and BODLEY 1981) together with the lack of a significant effect of the mutations at Glu-148 on the NAD glycohydrolysis reaction, which most likely occurs via an oxycarbonium intermediate, diminished the likelihood that ADP-ribosylation occurred by an S_N1-type reaction, thus leaving the other potential roles for glutamic acid to be considered.

3.2 A Possible Role for an Active-Site Histidine in Catalysis

The pH profiles for the wild-type DTA revealed the presence of a titratable group that was dramatically affected by the presence or absence of the carboxyl side chain (WILSON et al. 1990b). This group, which must be protonated for ADP-ribosylation to occur, since the reaction rate declined with increasing pH, exhibited an apparent pK_a of 6.2–6.3. Since this pK_a was above the normal range of pK_a values for the glutamic acid side-chain carboxyl group in proteins, it was considered unlikely that the observed titration was due to Glu-148, and a more complex explanation for the results was proposed, involving both Glu-148 and an active-site histidine at position 21. On the basis of independent evidence (PAPINI et al. 1989) that the single, highly conserved His-21 of DTA titrates with a pK_a value of 6.3, as determined from the pH dependence of both NAD binding and diethyl pyrocarbonate modification of His-21, it was proposed (WILSON et al. 1990b) that the observed kinetic titration probably represented the ionization of the His-21 side-chain imidazole and that substitution of glutamine or serine for Glu-148 strongly affected this titration. From the X-ray crystallographic structure of ETA (Fig. 3), it was inferred that the conserved histidine in ETA (His-440) corresponding to His-21 of DT lies within the active-site pocket (ALLURED et al. 1986; PAPINI et al. 1989). It was thus proposed (WILSON et al. 1990b) that both His-21 and Glu-148 may be involved in the catalysis of ADP-ribosylation, where the role of the carboxyl group of Glu-148 may be to maintain a particular active-site conformation necessary for catalysis to occur, such as confining the position of the imidazole ring of His-21. Or, alternatively, it may function to somehow influence the nucleophilicity of the incoming diphthamide through acid-base interaction with the histidine. Experiments designed to examine the role of His-21 by site-directed mutagenesis and biochemical analysis are currently in progress (BLANKE et al., unpublished work) and should yield insight into the reaction mechanism. Other experiments designed to determine the ionization state of the glutamic acid carboxyl group and the imidazole ring of the histidine by nuclear magnetic resonance (NMR) spectroscopy are also currently underway (BLANKE et al., unpublished work).

3.3 Effect of Carboxyl Side-Chain Position on Catalysis

While the enzymatic properties of DTA have been much more extensively studied than those of ETA, similar results from mutagenesis and biochemical analysis have been obtained for ETA. Recent studies on other mutations of ETA have given additional information about the active-site structure and the reaction mechanism. The dramatic effect of changing glutamic acid to aspartic acid at the active site in both DT and ETA suggested that the rate of reaction depends strongly on the position of the side-chain carboxyl group. Shortening of the side chain by one methylene unit evidently prevented the carboxyl group from effectively interacting with either or both substrates (TWETEN et al. 1985; DOUGLAS and COLLIER 1987, 1990; WILSON et al. 1990b). The placement of the glutamic acid side chain on a β-strand deep within the prominent active-site cleft of domain III in the crystal structure of ETA (Fig. 3) supports this notion (ALLURED et al. 1986). The effect that lengthening the side chain might have on enzyme activity was consequently investigated (LUKAC and COLLIER 1988b) by substituting Glu-553 with cysteine and derivatizing it with iodoacetic acid to create an engineered carboxyl-containing side chain that was approximately 1 Å longer than the side chain of glutamic acid. While the cysteine mutant was far less active ($<0.01\%$) than the wild-type ETA, carboxymethylation restored the enzymatic activity of the mutant protein to approximately one-sixth that of the wild-type toxin, demonstrating that the enzyme-substrate complex can accommodate the slightly longer *S*-carboxymethylcysteine side chain. On the other hand, carboxamidomethylation failed to reactivate the mutant toxin, in keeping with results obtained showing the importance of the acidic function of the carboxyl group in catalysis, where it was demonstrated that substitution of Glu-148 in DT or Glu-553 in ETA with uncharged, isosteric glutamine resulted in even further loss of enzymic activity than substitution with aspartic acid.

3.4 Other Active-Site Residues

Within the active-site cleft, near Glu-553 in the X-ray crystal structure of ETA (Fig. 3), are several conserved, aromatic amino acid residues, including two tyrosines and two tryptophans, that could potentially participate in substrate binding or catalysis. The phenolic hydroxyl groups of the two prominent, active-site tyrosine residues in ETA, Tyr-470 and Tyr-481, have been tested for their potential interactions with NAD and EF-2 by replacing each residue with phenylalanine (LUKAC and COLLIER 1988a). Mutating Tyr-470 to phenylalanine was found to cause no significant effect on either ADP-ribosyltransferase or NAD-glycohydrolase activity, implying that the phenolic hydroxyl of Tyr-470 is not directly involved in enzymic catalysis, although it may still play a role in hydrophobic stacking interactions with the aromatic rings of NAD. Substitution of phenylalanine for Tyr-481 similarly resulted in little or no change in toxin interactions with NAD or in NAD glycohydrolysis. However, there was about a ten-fold decrease in ADP-ribosyltransferase activity, suggesting that the phenolic hydroxyl of Tyr-481 may have a minor effect on EF-2 binding, active-site conformation, or some other aspect of catalysis. On the basis of sequence homology, the mutation of Tyr-54 and Tyr-65 in DT to phenylalanine would be expected to give similar results to those found for Tyr-470 and Tyr-481, respectively, in ETA.

Binding of NAD has been shown to quench the total intrinsic protein fluorescence of the catalytically active fragments of DT and ETA by up to 80% (KANDEL et al. 1974; CHUNG and COLLIER 1977a; LORY et al. 1980). This dramatic effect has been attributable to the perturbation of one or both of the two active-site tryptophans present in the catalytic domains of the toxins. Binding of NAD was also found to cause the appearance of a weak, broad absorbance band ($\lambda = 360$ nm, $\varepsilon = 500$), which was not observed with either toxin or NAD alone and which was postulated to represent a charge-transfer complex involving the nicotinamide ring of NAD with one or both of the tryptophans. Each of these tryptophans in DT, Trp-50 and Trp-153, have together or individually been replaced with phenylalanine to probe the role of each in binding and catalysis and to better understand the interactions underlying the fluorescence and absorbance changes upon NAD binding. Preliminary data (WILSON et al., unpublished work) indicate that the single and double mutations still retain some ADP-ribosyltransferase and NAD-glycohydrolase activity and that binding of NAD appears to be somewhat affected. More precise analysis of the enzymatic and optical properties of the purified mutant proteins is currently in progress.

4 Models for Binding of NAD to the Active Site

Because of the significant degree of sequence similarity at the active-site pocket of the catalytic domains in DT and ETA, computer-based moleculer modeling, using distance geometry and energy minimization programs, has recently been used (DOMENIGHINI et al. 1991) to fit the enzymic domain of DT into the coordinate set of domain III of native ETA. The results from these modeling studies indicate that the two toxins share overall folding and organizational patterns in their catalytic domains and that they are virtually superimposable at the NAD-binding pocket, while their differences are confined to the protein surface. Thus, using the three-dimensional X-ray crystal structure of ETA as a template, two models for NAD binding at the active sites of ETA and DT have been proposed (BRANDHUBER et al. 1988; DOMENIGHINI et al. 1991). Because of the similar size and aromatic character of the nicotinamide and adenine rings of NAD, it was found that the NAD molecule could be fitted into the active-site cleft of these toxins in two equally favorable, yet opposite, orientations. Consistent with the possible models are the results from recent photolabeling experiments, in which Tyr-65 of DT was photolabeled by both 8-azidoadenine and 8-azidoadenosine (PAPINI et al. 1991). The competitive inhibitors adenine, adenosine, and nicotinamide (KANDEL et al. 1974) appeared to bind to the same portions of the active site, since all three inhibitors strongly reduced the extent of photolabeling by the azido derivatives.

The first model proposed (BRANDHUBER et al. 1988) that the NAD molecule fits into the cleft with the adenine ring bound in the hydrophobic pocket defined by the aromatic rings of the two tyrosines, Tyr-470 and Tyr-481 in ETA, corresponding to Tyr-54 and Tyr-65 in DT, respectively, and the nicotinamide ring stacked against the aromatic ring of Trp-466 in ETA, or Trp-50 in DT. Alternatively, NAD could also be fitted in the opposite orientation with the adenine ring in contact with the tryptophan and the nicotinamide ring near the tyrosines. It has recently been proposed (DOMENIGHINI et al. 1991) that the second model may better account for the available experimental data, including the photolabeling results at both Tyr-65 and Glu-148 in DT, and Glu-553 in ETA, and the observed enzymatic properties of the toxins, and may provide somewhat more favorable hydrophobic stacking interactions for the aromatic rings, resulting in tighter NAD binding.

The existence of these two possible modes for NAD binding illustrates the flexible structure of the active site, as was shown by its ability to accommodate the longer *S*-carboxymethylcysteine side chain at position 148. Recently, further evidence of the remarkably flexible nature of the catalytic domain has been obtained. During the course of studies designed to construct mutant forms of DT and ETA that would be suitable for introduction as toxoids into a live multivalent vaccine, the effects of specific deletions of various active-site residues have been examined in both toxins (KILLEEN and COLLIER, submitted for publication). As had been previously found for the Glu-553 deletion mutant of ETA, the deletion of the corresponding Glu-148 in DT virtually abolished (by $>10^5$-fold) both ADP-ribosyltransferase activity and cytotoxicity.

In both toxin models, the critical active-site glutamic acid lies on a β-strand at the back of a hydrophobic pocket defining part of the active site. This β-strand is connected to an adjacent β-strand, ending at the conserved residue Glu-547 in ETA or Glu-142 in DT, by a small loop segment of hydrophilic amino acids. The loop, comprised of residues 548–551 in ETA and residues 143–146 in DT, protrudes toward the protein's surface, away from the active-site pocket, and could not be traced in the ETA crystal structure because it was too flexible to be resolved.

5 Deletion of an Active-Site Loop Flanking the Catalytic Glutamic Acid

When one or more of the amino acids in the loop flanking the active-site Glu-148 in DT were independently deleted (KILLEEN and COLLIER, submitted for publication), both the individual amino acid deletions and the multiple amino acid deletions caused no major alterations in protein expression, stability, or immunoreactivity. Nevertheless, all of the mutant toxins, lacking a glutamic acid adjacent to Tyr-149, were found to exhibit no detectable ADP-ribosyltransferase activity ($<10^{-4}$ that of wild-type toxin). Although less extensively studied, similar results have been obtained for mutants of ETA containing deletions of the two residues flanking Glu-553.

Surprisingly, as long as a glutamic acid was positioned next to Tyr-149 in DT, deletion of any or all of the amino acids comprising the loop segment still allowed the active site to retain a significant degree of its appropriate, active conformation such that the glutamic acid could function in catalysis, albeit to a somewhat lesser extent. The activities of the mutants having deletions amino-proximal to Glu-148 generally ranged from 0.5%–10% that of the wild-type toxin; the small differences in the amount of retention apparently depending on whether the carboxyl side chain favored an orientation on the β-strand such that it could effectively interact with the reaction substrates. On the other hand, replacing the conserved Glu-142 at the opposite end of the loop segment in DT (WILSON and COLLIER, unpublished work), corresponding to Glu-547 in ETA, with other amino acids, such as alanine, aspartic acid, glutamine, or serine, had no apparent effect on the toxin's enzymic activity. Thus, the pliable, active-site segment, defined by residues 141–149, corresponding to residues 546–554 in ETA, contains a remarkably flexible loop, which can be shortened significantly in length and yet still allow the toxin to retain a substantial amount of its enzymic activity.

6 Future Prospects and Concluding Remarks

Although the studies of the other active-site residues mentioned above are incomplete, all the evidence accumulated to date indicates that the acitve-site glutamic acids, Glu-148 in DT, Glu-553 in ETA, and Glu-129 in PT, are by far the most sensitive to mutation, and so, appear to be the most important for catalysis of ADP-ribosylation. Interpretation of the combined results from mutagenesis and biochemical analyses, as well as molecular modeling, may be facilitated once the detailed, three-dimensional structure of DTA has been obtained. X-ray crystallographic studies of the dimeric form of whole DT (COLLIER et al. 1982; MCKEEVER and SARMA 1982; KANTARDJIEFF et al. 1987) and of DTA (KANTARDJIEFF et al. 1989) are currently underway and should yield valuable information toward the understanding of the relationship between the two toxins and their active sites.

Recently, a new activity has been attributed to DT by a group of researchers. This group has reported that certain toxin-treated target cells undergo extensive DNA fragmentation prior to cytolysis (CHANG et al. 1989b). Furthermore, the DNase activity responsible was reported to be a property of the toxin itself (CHANG et al. 1989a; LESSNICK et al. 1990), residing specifically within the catalytic A fragment (CHANG et al. 1989a; NAKAMURA and WISNIESKI 1990; BRUCE et al. 1990; LESSNICK et al. 1990). Other researchers have not been able to substantiate this report, however, and have presented (BODLEY 1990; JOHNSON 1990; WILSON et al. 1990a) evidence that the reported nuclease activity may represent an artifact due to a contaminating DNase present in partially purified toxin preparations.

An important question raised by all of these studies is whether the active-site glutamic acid will prove to be a common, important feature of ADP-ribosylation among all ADP-ribosyltransferases. The catalytic S-1 subunit of PT has recently been found to contain an analogous, catalytically important glutamic acid at position 129; however, when the glutamic acids were aligned, very little sequence homology was found between the S-1 subunit of PT and DTA or ETA (BARBIERI et al. 1989). S-1 does share some homology with cholera toxin (CT), but the residue in CT corresponding to Glu-129 in S-1 is a tryptophan (Trp-127). Although further studies are needed, it may be possible that the topology of the active sites might be such that another amino acid carboxyl group is nearby and can play an analogous role in catalysis for the other ADP-ribosylating proteins. However, it should be reiterated that there is another consistent feature among all these toxins, namely the presence of a unique, active-site histidine residue, which could conceivably function in conjunction with the carboxyl group to catalyze the ADP-ribosyltransfer reaction. Studies by several research groups are currently in progress to resolve these issues and to address the broader question of the evolutionary relationships among these ADP-ribosyltransferases.

References

Allured VS, Collier RJ, Carroll SF, McKay DB (1986) Structure of exotoxin A of *Pseudomonas aeruginosa* at 3.0-Angstrom resolution. Proc Natl Acad Sci USA 83: 1320–1324

Allured VS, Brandhuber BJ, McKay DB (1987) Structure and mechanism of exotoxin A of *Pseudomonas aeruginosa*. In: Bonavida B, Collier RJ (eds) Membrane-mediated cytotoxicity. Liss, New York, pp 3–7

Barbieri JT, Collier RJ (1987) Expression of a mutant, full-length form of diphtheria toxin in *Escherichia coli*. Infect Immun 55: 1647–1651

Barbieri JT, Mende-Mueller LM, Rappuoli R, Collier RJ (1989) Photolabeling of Glu-129 of the S-1 subunit of pertussis toxin with NAD. Infect Immun 57: 3549–3554

Bodley JW (1990) Does diphtheria toxin have nuclease activity? Science 250: 832–838

Brandhuber BJ, Allured VS, Falbel TG, McKay DB (1988) Mapping of the enzymatic active site of *Pseudomonas aeruginosa* exotoxin A. Proteins Struct Funct Genet 3: 146–154

Bruce C, Baldwin RL, Lessnick SL, Wisnieski BJ (1990) Diphtheria toxin and its ADP-ribosyltransferase-defective homologue CRM197 possess deoxy-ribonuclease activity. Proc Natl Acad Sci USA 87: 2995–2998

Carroll SF, Collier RJ (1984) NAD binding site of diphtheria toxin: identification of a residue within the nicotinamide subsite by photochemical modification with NAD. Proc Natl Acad Sci USA 81: 3307–3311

Carroll SF, Collier RJ (1987) Active site of *Pseudomonas aeruginosa* exotoxin A: glumatic acid 553 is photolabeled by NAD and shows functional homology with glutamic acid 148 of diphtheria toxin. J Biol Chem 262: 8707–8711

Carroll SF, Collier RJ (1988) Amino acid sequence homology between the enzymic domains of diphtheria toxin and *Pseudomonas aeruginosa* exotoxin A. Mol Microbiol 2: 293–296

Carroll SF, McCloskey JA, Crain PF, Oppenheimer NJ, Marschner TM, Collier RJ (1985) Photoaffinity labeling of diphtheria toxin fragment A with NAD: structure of the photoproduct at position 148. Proc Natl Acad Sci USA 82: 7237–7241

Chang MP, Baldwin RL, Bruce C, Wisnieski BJ (1989a) Second cytotoxic pathway of diphtheria toxin suggested by nuclease activity. Science 246: 1165–1168

Chang MP, Bramhall J, Graves S, Bonavida B, Wisnieski BJ (1989b) Internucleosomal DNA cleavage precedes diphtheria toxin-induced cytolysis: evidence that cell lysis is not a simple consequence of translation inhibition. J Biol Chem 264: 15261–15267

Chung DW, Collier RJ (1977a) Enzymatically active peptide from the adenosine diphosphate-ribosylating toxin of *Pseudomonas aeruginosa*. Infect Immun 16: 832–841

Chung DW, Collier RJ (1977b) The mechanism of ADP-ribosylation of elongation factor 2 catalyzed by fragment A from diphtheria toxin. Biochim Biophys Acta 483: 248–257

Cieplak W, Locht C, Mar VL, Burnette WN, Keith JM (1990) Photolabeling of mutant forms of the S1 subunit of pertussis toxin with NAD. Biochem J 268: 547–551

Cockle SA (1989) Identification of an active-site residue in subunit S1 of pertussis toxin by photocrosslinking to NAD. FEBS Lett 249: 329–332

Collier RJ (1975) Diphtheria toxin: mode of action and structure. Bacteriol Rev 39: 54–85

Collier RJ (1982) Structure and activity of diphtheria toxin. In: Hayaishi O, Ueda K (eds) ADP-ribosylation reactions. Academic, New York, pp 575–592

Collier RJ, Kandel J (1971) Structure and activity of diphtheria toxin. I. Thiol-dependent dissociation of a fraction of toxin into enzymically active and inactive fragments. J Biol Chem 246: 1496–1503

Collier RJ, Westbrook EM, McKay DB, Eisenberg D (1982) X-ray grade crystals of diphtheria toxin. J Biol Chem 257: 5283–5285

Domenighini M, Montecucco C, Ripka WC, Rappuoli R (1991) Computer modeling of the NAD binding site of ADP-ribosylating toxins: common active site and possible mechanism of catalysis. Mol Microbiol (in press)

Douglas CD, Collier RJ (1987) Exotoxin A of *Pseudomonas aeruginosa*: substitution of glutamic acid 553 with aspartic acid drastically reduces toxicity and enzymatic activity. J Bacteriol 169: 4967–4971

Douglas CM, Collier RJ (1990) *Pseudomonas aeruginosa* exotoxin A: alterations of biological and biochemical properties resulting from mutation of glumatic acid 553 to aspartic acid. Biochemistry 29: 5043–5049

Drazin R, Kandel J, Collier RJ (1971) Structure and activity of diphtheria toxin. II. Attack by trypsin at a specific site within the intact toxin molecule. J Biol Chem 246: 1504–1510

Eidels L, Proia RL, Hart DA (1983) Membrane receptors for bacterial toxins. Microbiol Rev 47: 596–620

Gill DM (1988) Sequence homologies among the enzymically active portions of ADP-ribosylating toxins. In: Fehrenback FE, Alouf JE, Falmagne P, Goebel W, Jeljaszewicz J, Jurgens D, Rappuoli R (eds) Bacterial protein toxins, 3 European Workshop. Fischer, New York, pp 315–323

Gill DM, Pappenheimer AM Jr (1971) Structure-activity relationships in diphtheria toxin. J Biol Chem 246: 1492–1495

Gill DM, Pappenheimer AM Jr, Brown R, Kurnick JT (1969) Studies on the mode of action of diphtheria toxin. VII. Toxin-stimulated hydrolysis of nicotinamide adenine dinucleotide in mammalian cell extracts. J Exp Med 129: 1–21

Gray GL, Smith DH, Baldridge JS, Harkins RN, Vasil ML, Chen EY, Heyneker HL (1984) Cloning, nucleotide sequence, and expression in *Escherichia coli* of the exotoxin A structural gene of *Pseudomonas aeruginosa*. Proc Natl Acad Sci USA 81: 2645–2649

Greenfield L, Bjorn MJ, Horn G, Fong D, Buck GA, Collier RJ, Kaplan DA (1983) Nucleotide sequence of the structural gene for diphtheria toxin carried by corynebacteriophage beta. Proc Natl Acad Sci USA 80: 6853–6857

Honjo T, Nishizuka Y, Hayaishi O (1968) Diphtheria toxin-dependent adenosine diphosphate ribosylation of aminoacyl transferase II and inhibition of protein synthesis. J Biol Chem 243: 3553–3555

Honjo T, Nishizuka Y, Hayaishi O (1969) Adenosine diphosphoribosylation of aminoacyl transferase II by diphtheria toxin. Cold Spring Harbor Symp Quant Biol 34: 603–608

Iglewski BH, Kabat D (1975) NAD-dependent inhibition of protein synthesis by *Pseudomonas aeruginosa* toxin. Proc Natl Acad Sci USA 72: 2284–2288

Iglewski BH, Liu PV, Kabat D (1977) Mechanism of action of *Pseudomonas aeruginosa* exotoxin A: adenosine diphosphate-ribosylation of mammalian elongation factor 2 in vitro and in vivo. Infect Immun 15: 138–144

Jacobson MK, Jacobson EL (eds) (1989) ADP-ribose transfer reactions. Mechanisms and biological significance. Springer, Berlin Heidelberg New York

Johnson VG (1990) Does diphtheria toxin have nuclease activity? Science 250: 832–838

Kandel J, Collier RJ, Chung DW (1974) Interaction of fragment A from diphtheria toxin with nicotinamide adenine dinucleotide. J Biol Chem 249: 2088–2097

Kantardjieff K, Dijkstra B, Westbrook EM, Barbieri JT, Carroll SF, Collier RJ, Eisenberg D (1987) Structural studies of diphtheria toxin. In: Oxender D (ed) Protein structure, folding, and design 2. Liss, New York, pp187–200

Kantardjieff K, Collier RJ, Eisenberg D (1989) X-ray grade crystals of the enzymatic fragment of diphtheria toxin. J Biol Chem 264: 10402–10404

Leppla SH, Martin OC, Muehl LA (1978) The exotoxin of *P. aeruginosa*: a proenzyme having an unusual mode of activation. Biochem Biophys Res Commun 81: 532–538

Lessnick SL, Bruce C, Baldwin RL, Chang MP, Nakamura LT, Wisnieski BJ (1990) Does diphtheria toxin have nuclease activity? Science 250: 832–838

Lory S, Collier RJ (1980) Expression of enzymic activity by exotoxin A from *Pseudomonas aeruginosa*. Infect Immun 28: 494–501

Lory S, Carroll SF, Bernard PD, Collier RJ (1980) Ligand interactions of diphtheria toxin. I. Binding and hydrolysis of NAD. J Biol Chem 255: 12011–12015

Lukac M, Collier RJ (1988a) *Pseudomonas aeruginosa* exotoxin A: effects of mutating tyrosine-470 and tyrosine-481 to phenylalanine. Biochemistry 27: 7629–7632

Lukac M, Collier RJ (1988b) Restoration of enzymic activity and cytotoxicity of mutant, E553C, *Pseudomonas aeruginosa* exotoxin A by reaction with iodoacetic acid. J Biol Chem 263: 6146–6149

Lukac M, Pier GB, Collier RJ (1988) Toxoid of *Pseudomonas aeruginosa* exotoxin A generated by deletion of an active-site residue. Infect Immun 56: 3095–3098

McKeever B, Sarma R (1982) Preliminary crystallographic investigation of the protein toxin from *Corynebacterium diphtheriae*. J Biol Chem 257: 6923–6925

Middlebrook JL, Dorland RB (1977a) Differential chemical protection of mammalian cells from the exotoxins of *Corynebacterium diphtheriae* and *Pseudomonas aeruginosa*. Infect Immun 16: 232–239

Middlebrook JL, Dorland RB (1977b) Response of cultured mammalian cells to the exotoxins of *Pseudomonas aeruginosa* and *Corynebacterium diphtheriae*: differential cytotoxicity. Can J Microbiol 23: 183–189

Moss J, Vaughan M (1990) ADP-ribosylating toxins and G proteins. Insights into signal transduction. American Society for Microbiology, Washington, DC

Nakamura LT, Wisnieski BJ (1990) Characterization of the deoxyribonuclease activity of diphtheria toxin. J Biol Chem 265: 5237–5241

Oppenheimer NJ, Bodley JW (1981) Diphtheria toxin: site and configuration of ADP-ribosylation 'diphthamide' in elongation factor 2. J Biol Chem 256: 8579–8581

Papini E, Schiavo G, Sandona D, Rappuoli R, Montecucco C (1989) Histidine 21 is at the NAD binding site of diphtheria toxin. J Biol chem 264: 12385–12388

Papini E, Santucci A, Schiavo G, Domenighini M, Neri P, Rappuoli R, Montecucco C (1991) Tyrosine 65 is photolabeled by 8-azidoadenine and 8-azidoadenosine at the NAD binding site of diphtheria toxin. J Biol Chem 266: 2494–2498

Pappenheimer AM Jr (1977) Diphtheria toxin. Annu Rev Biochem 46: 69–94

Pizza M, Bartoloni A, Prugnola A, Silvestri S, Rappuoli R (1988) Subunit S1 of pertussis toxin:

mapping of the regions essential for ADP-ribosyltransferase activity. Proc Natl Acad Sci USA 85: 7521–7525

Sadoff JC, Buck GA, Iglewski BH, Bjorn MJ, Groman NB (1982) Immunological cross-reactivity in the absence of DNA homology between *Pseudomonas* toxin A and diphtheria toxin. Infect Immun 37: 250–254

Tweten RK, Barbieri JT, Collier RJ (1985) Diphtheria toxin: effect of substituting aspartic acid for glutamic acid 148 on ADP-ribosyltransferase activity. J Biol Chem 260: 10392–10394

Van Ness BG, Howard JB, Bodley JW (1980a) ADP-ribosylation of elongation factor 2 by diphtheria toxin: isolation and properties of the novel ribosyl-amino acid and its hydrolysis products. J Biol Chem 255: 10717–10720

Van Ness BG, Howard JB, Bodley JW (1980b) ADP-ribosylation of elongation factor 2 by diphtheria toxin. NMR spectra and proposed structures of 'ribosyl-diphthamide' and its hydrolysis products. J Biol Chem 255: 10710–10716

Vasil ML, Iglewski BH (1978) Comparative toxicities of diphtheria toxin and *Pseudomonas aeruginosa* exotoxin A: evidence for different cell receptors. J Gen Microbiol 108: 333–337

Vasill ML, Iglewski BH (1978) Comparative toxicities of diphtheria toxin and *Pseudomonas aeruginosa*. Infect Immun 16: 353–361

Wilson BA, Blanke SR, Murphy JR, Pappenheimer AM Jr, Collier RJ (1990a) Does diphtheria toxin have nuclease activity? Science 250: 832–838

Wilson BA, Reich KA, Weinstein BR, Collier RJ (1990b) Active-site mutations of diphtheria toxin: effects of replacing glutamic acid-148 with aspartic acid, glutamine, or serine. Biochemistry 29: 8643–8651

Zhao JM, London E (1988) Localization of the active site of diphtheria toxin. Biochemistry 27: 3398–3403

Enhancement of Cholera Toxin-Catalyzed ADP-Ribosylation by Guanine Nucleotide-Binding Proteins

I. M. SERVENTI, J. MOSS, and M. VAUGHAN

1 Activation of Adenylyl Cyclase by Cholera Toxin

Cholera toxin binds to the membrane of intestinal mucosal cells and activates adenylyl cyclase (KIMBERG et al. 1971). The resultant increase in cyclic AMP and possibly other factors leads to the pathological disturbances in fluid and electrolyte flux observed in clinical cholera (BIRNBAUMER et al. 1990; FINKELSTEIN 1973; KELLY 1986; MOSS and VAUGHAN 1988a; PETERSON and OCHOA 1989). *Vibrio cholerae* secretes cholera toxin as an 84-kDa oligomeric protein composed of one A ($\sim$27 kDa) and five B ($\sim$11 kDa) subunits (GILL 1976a, 1977); the A subunit is proteolytically nicked to produce two polypeptides, A1 ($\sim$21 kDa) and A2 ($\sim$6 kDa) (GILL and RAPPAPORT 1979), linked through a disulfide bond that on reduction generates the enzymatically active A1 protein (GILL and KING 1975; MEKALANOS et al. 1979b; MOSS et al. 1979c). Intoxication of cells requires intact holotoxin; the B subunits are responsible for toxin binding to the membrane (CUATRECASAS 1973 a, b, c; HOLMGREN et al. 1973, 1974; VAN HEYNINGEN et al. 1971) via specific interaction with the oligosaccharide moiety of the monosialoganglioside G_{M1} (galactosyl-*N*-acetylgalactosaminyl-[*N*-acetylneuraminyl]-galactosylglucosylceramide) (FISHMAN et al. 1978; SATTLER et al. 1978; SCHWARZMANN et al. 1978).

Laboratory of Cellular Metabolism, National Heart, Lung, and Blood Institute, National Institutes of Health, Bethesda, MD 20892, USA

Current Topics in Microbiology and Immunology, Vol. 175

Cholera toxin activation of adenylyl cyclase requires NAD (GILL 1975). In vitro the isolated A protomer (A1–A2) catalyzes hydrolysis of NAD to ADP-ribose and nicotinamide (Table 1, reaction 1; MOSS et al. 1976) and transfer of the ADP-ribose moiety to arginine (Table 1, reaction 2; MOSS and VAUGHAN 1977a) demonstrating that cholera toxin is an enzyme possessing both NAD^+ glycohydrolase (NADase) and ADP-ribosyltransferase activities. In vitro cholera toxin also catalyzes the ADP-ribosylation of other simple guanidino compounds, such as agmatine (MEKALANOS et al. 1979a; MOSS and VAUGHAN 1977a; MOSS et al. 1979c), and nonspecific protein substrates, such as lysozyme and histones (Table 1, reaction 3; MOSS and VAUGHAN 1978), as well as the auto-ADP-ribosylation of the toxin A1 subunit (Table 1, reaction 4; MOSS et al. 1980; TREPEL et al. 1977). The NADase and ADP-ribosyltransferase activities of cholera toxin are intrinsic to the thiol-activated A1 protein (MOSS et al. 1979c).

In a search to find a native substrate, several laboratories independently showed that a 42- to 45-kDa protein was ADP-ribosylated by cholera toxin in erythrocyte ghosts (CASSEL and PFEUFFER 1978; GILL and MEREN 1978) and S49 mouse lymphoma cell membranes (JOHNSON et al. 1978). A minor 52-kDa ADP-ribosylated species was also noted (JOHNSON et al. 1978). The incorporation of ADP-ribose into these proteins correlated with an increase in adenylyl cyclase activity (CASSEL and PFEUFFER 1978; GILL and MEREN 1978), was stimulated by GTP (GILL and MEREN 1978), was absent in membranes of S49 cyc^- mutant cells that lack GTP regulation of adenylyl cyclase (JOHNSON et al. 1978), and was not observed in membranes of S49 wild-type cells previously treated with cholera toxin (JOHNSON et al. 1978). All of these data suggested that in vivo toxin-catalyzed ADP-ribosylation was linked to adenylyl cyclase activation through G_S, the stimulatory guanine nucleotide-binding protein of the adenylyl cyclase system. These findings were further substantiated when NORTHUP et al. (1980) demonstrated that the 45- and 52-kDa α subunits of purified G_S ($G_{s\alpha}$) were indeed toxin substrates (Table 1, reaction 5).

Although activation of adenylyl cyclase by cholera toxin was dependent on NAD (GILL 1975), persistence of the activated state was NAD-independent (GILL 1976b). Solubilized systems revealed other requirements which contributed to understanding the underlying mechanism of toxin activation of adenylyl cyclase. GTP was necessary for toxin activation of adenylyl cyclase (CASSEL

Table 1. Enzymatic activities of cholera toxin A1 protein

No.	Reaction
1	$NAD + H_2O \rightarrow$ ADP-ribose + nicotinamide + H^+
2	NAD + arginine[1] $\rightarrow$ ADP-ribosylarginine + nicotinamide + H^+
3	NAD + (arginine)protein $\rightarrow$ ADP-ribosyl(arginine)protein + nicotinamide + H^+
4	NAD + CT-A1 $\rightarrow$ ADP-ribosyl-CT-A1 + nicotinamide + H^+
5	$NAD + G_{s\alpha} \rightarrow$ ADP-ribosyl-$G_{s\alpha}$ + nicotinamide + H^+

CT-A1, cholera toxin A1 protein

[1] Arginine or simple guanidino compounds, e.g., agmatine

and SELINGER 1977; ENOMOTO and GILL 1979, 1980; LIN et al. 1978; MOSS and VAUGHAN 1977b; NAKAYA et al. 1980) and for toxin-catalyzed ADP-ribosylation of the ~45- and 52-kDa membrane proteins (ENOMOTO and GILL 1980) now known to arise from splice variants of $G_{s\alpha}$ (BRAY et al. 1986; KOZASA et al. 1988; ROBISHAW et al. 1986b). G_s is the regulatory G protein identified by its ability to stimulate adenylyl cyclase in the presence of GTP or a nonhydrolyzable GTP analogue. It is a heterotrimer composed of α, β, and γ subunits. $G_{s\alpha}$ binds and hydrolyzes GTP; its GTP-bound form activates adenylyl cyclase and Ca^{2+} channels (for review see BIRNBAUMER et al. 1987; CASEY and GILMAN 1988; GILMAN 1987; MATTERA et al. 1989; YATANI et al. 1988). Its intrinsic GTPase activity hydrolyzes GTP to produce an inactive $G_{s\alpha}$·GDP form (BIRNBAUMER et al. 1987; CASEY and GILMAN 1988; GILMAN 1987). CASSEL and SELINGER (1977) originally proposed that toxin-catalyzed ADP-ribosylation of $G_{s\alpha}$ reduced its GTPase activity, thereby preserving the active $G_{s\alpha}$·GTP form, resulting in persistent activation of adenylyl cyclase. Consistent with this model is the observation that toxin-catalyzed ADP-ribosylation increased the sensitivity of adenylyl cyclase to GTP (GILL 1976b; LIN et al. 1978; NAKAYA et al. 1980). Toxin-catalyzed ADP-ribosylation also promoted dissociation of $G_{s\alpha}$ from $G_{\beta\gamma}$ (KAHN and GILMAN 1984b) and stimulated release of guanine nucleotide from membranes, thus opening up the site for GTP binding and promoting reactivation (BURNS et al. 1982, 1983).

Cholera toxin also catalyzes the ADP-ribosylation of the α subunit of G_t, the retinal G protein transducin, which activates a cyclic GMP phosphodiesterase (ABOOD et al. 1982; NAVON and FUNG 1984; STRYER and BOURNE 1986; VAN DOP et al. 1984) and G_{olf}, the olfactory G_s-like G protein, which activates olfactory adenylyl cyclase (JONES et al. 1990). ADP-ribosylation correlated with decreased GTP hydrolysis by $G_{t\alpha}$ (ABOOD et al. 1982; NAVON and FUNG 1984) and constitutive activation of G_{olf} (JONES et al. 1990). Using artificial substrates, MOSS and VAUGHAN (1977a) characterized cholera toxin as an NAD: arginine ADP-ribosyltransferase. Consistent with these findings VAN DOP et al. (1984) identified an arginine as the site of toxin-catalyzed ADP-ribosylation in $G_{t\alpha}$, later determined to be Arg-174 in $G_{t\alpha1}$ (MEDYNSKI et al. 1985; TANABE et al. 1985; YATSUNAMI and KHORANA 1985) and Arg-178 in $G_{t\alpha2}$ (LOCHRIE et al. 1985) based on the deduced amino acid sequences derived from their respective cDNA sequences and the peptide sequence of VAN DOP et al. (1984). Extrapolation of these data to $G_{s\alpha}$ pinpointed Arg-187 and Arg-201 as the respective sites of cholera toxin-catalyzed ADP-ribosylation in the 45- and 52-kDa forms of $G_{s\alpha}$ (JONES and REED 1987; ROBISHAW et al. 1986a).

$G_{s\alpha}$ mutational studies (BOURNE et al. 1989; FREISSMUTH and GILMAN 1989; LANDIS et al. 1989) support the hypothesis that this site is essential for regulating the intrinsic "timing device" of GTP hydrolysis, but raise some question as to whether this specific arginine is the only site of cholera toxin-catalyzed ADP-ribosylation. Replacement of Arg-187 in the 45-kDa $G_{s\alpha}$ variant with Ala, Glu, or Lys (FREISSMUTH and GILMAN 1989) and Arg-201 in the 52-kDa $G_{s\alpha}$ variant with Cys of His (BOURNE et al. 1989; LANDIS et al. 1989) resulted in mutant proteins with greatly reduced rates of GTP hydrolysis (30- to 100-fold lower than wild type) which constitutively activated adenylyl cyclase in the presence of GTP. Surprisingly, toxin-catalyzed ADP-ribosylation of the mutant $G_{s\alpha}$ proteins was not completely abolished, but greatly reduced (10%–30% of wild type). Whether this indicates that the site of ADP-ribosylation is not Arg-187 in the 45-kDa $G_{s\alpha}$ species or Arg-201 in the 53-kDa $G_{s\alpha}$ species is unclear but may simply mean that if the preferred site is not available the toxin will use another arginine. There are several arginines in the vicinity that could serve as ADP-ribose acceptors (JONES and REED 1987; ROBISHAW et al. 1986a).

Activation of adenylyl cyclase by cholera toxin is persistent, and ADP-ribosylation of $G_{s\alpha}$ appears to be irreversible (CHANG et al. 1983; O'KEEFE and CUATRECASAS 1974). No correlation has been established between the reversal of toxin activation of adenylyl cyclase and the presence of cellular ADP-ribosylarginine hydrolase activity (MOSS et al. 1985). Exposure of GH_3 pituitary cells to cholera toxin resulted in persistent activation of adenylyl cyclase and increased degradation of ADP-ribosylated $G_{s\alpha}$ (CHANG and BOURNE 1989). $G_{s\alpha}$ degradation did not correlate with a loss in adenylyl cyclase activity as might be expected if the amount of $G_{s\alpha}$ were limiting; it proceeded by an undefined, nonlysosomal, cAMP-independent mechanism. The authors concluded that ADP-ribosylation marked $G_{s\alpha}$ for degradation (CHANG and BOURNE 1989). Whether this degradation mechanism plays a role in reversing intoxication by cholera toxin is unknown. Although cholera toxin remained bound to fibroblast membranes for a time on the order of days (CHANG et al. 1983), levels of immunoreactive $G_{s\alpha}$ in the GH_3 cells decreased by 74%–95% in 8 h (CHANG and BOURNE 1989).

2 ADP-Ribosylation Factors (ARFs): Proteins that Stimulate the ADP-Ribosyltransferase Activities of Cholera Toxin

2.1 Biochemical Properties of ARFs

Several membrane and soluble protein cofactors from a variety of sources were identified by their ability to enhance cholera toxin activation of adenylyl cyclase and/or toxin-catalyzed ADP-ribosylation (ENOMOTO and ASAKAWA 1982; ENOMOTO and GILL 1979, 1980; GILL 1976b; GILL and COBURN 1987; GILL and MEREN 1978, 1983; GILL and WOOLKALIS 1988; GRAVES et al. 1983; KAHN and GILMAN 1984a; LEVINE and CUATRECASAS 1981; PINKETT and ANDERSON 1982; SCHLEIFER et al. 1982; SCHMIDT et al. 1987; TSAI et al. 1987, 1988; WOOLKALIS et al. 1988). Although the properties of these factors differed somewhat, most were small (~11–21 kDa) (ENOMOTO and ASAKAWA 1982; ENOMOTO and GILL 1979, 1980; KAHN and GILMAN 1984a; LEVINE and CUATRECASAS 1981; PINKETT and ANDERSON

1982; SCHLEIFER et. al. 1982; SCHMIDT et al. 1987; TSAI et al. 1987, 1988) and were heat-labile and/or trypsin-sensitive (ENOMOTO and ASAKAWA 1982; ENOMOTO and GILL 1979; KAHN and GILMAN 1984a; LEVINE and CUATRECASAS 1981; SCHLEIFER et al. 1982). In all cases, optimal conditions for toxin-catalyzed activation of adenylyl cyclase or ADP-ribosylation required, in addition to activated toxin, NAD and a nucleoside triphosphate, initially thought to be ATP (GILL 1976b; GILL and MEREN 1978; LEVINE and CUATRECASAS 1981) but later found to be GTP (ENOMOTO and GILL 1979, 1980) or a nonhydrolyzable GTP analogue (ENOMOTO and GILL 1980).

KAHN and GILMAN (1984a) purified a membrane-associated ADP-ribosylation factor (mARF), which migrated as a doublet of ~21 kDa on denaturing polyacrylamide gels and required both sodium dodecyl sulfate (SDS) and cholate for stability. mARF was later shown to bind guanine nucleotides with high affinity (KAHN and GILMAN 1986); ARF·GTP was the active species, whereas ARF·GDP did not support stimulation of cholera toxin-catalyzed modification of $G_{s\alpha}$ as measured by reconstitution of modified $G_{s\alpha}$ with adenylyl cyclase in cyc^- cell membranes (KAHN and GILMAN 1986) or ADP-ribosylation of the α subunit of purified G_s (TSAI et al. 1987). Nonhydrolyzable analogues of GTP, but not GDP or ATP, were capable of stimulating the ADP-ribosyltransferase activities of cholera toxin in the presence of mARF (TSAI et al. 1987). No ARF GTPase activity was detected although ARF was isolated with ~0.9 mol of bound GDP per mole of ARF (KAHN and GILMAN 1986). In yeast cell extracts an ARF GTPase-activating protein (GAP), as was found for Ras (TRAHEY and MCCORMICK 1987), was observed (STEARNS et al. 1990a). No ARF-related GTP/GDP exchange factors have been identified. The cytosolic factor (CF) of GILL and coworkers (ENOMOTO and GILL 1980; GILL and COBURN 1987; GILL and MEREN 1983; WOOLKALIS et al. 1988), originally proposed to be a GTP/GDP exchange factor, immunologically cross-reacted with antibodies against mARF (KAHN et al. 1988) and is most likely a cytosolic form of ARF, whereas the S factor (GILL and COBURN 1987; GILL and MEREN 1983) is likely to be mARF (GILL and COBURN 1987; KAHN et al. 1988).

Despite the fact that ARF was first purified from membranes, immunological data indicated that 50%–90% of ARF was soluble (KAHN et al. 1988). TSAI et al. (1988) purified two cytosolic forms of ARF (sARFI and sARFII) from bovine brain. Like mARF, the soluble ARFs are ~20-kDa proteins that in the presence of GTP or a nonhydrolyzable GTP analogue stimulate the NAD glycohydrolase activity and all of the ADP-ribosyltransferase activities of cholera toxin (Table 1; TSAI et al. 1988). In the presence of GTP, ARF stimulated the toxin-catalyzed ADP-ribosylation of numerous membrane and cytosolic proteins, as well as the toxin A1 protein and ARF itself (TSAI et al. 1987, 1988). In the presence of cholate, toxin-catalyzed ADP-ribosylation of $G_{s\alpha}$ was greatly enhanced by dimyristoylphosphatidylcholine (DMPC) (SCHLEIFER et al. 1982). The effect of DMPC/cholate varied, however, with the specific substrate or specific cholera toxin ADP-ribosyltransferase activity being measured (SCHLEIFER et al. 1982; TSAI et al. 1987, 1988). sARF-stimulated, GTP-dependent toxin-catalyzed ADP-ribosylation

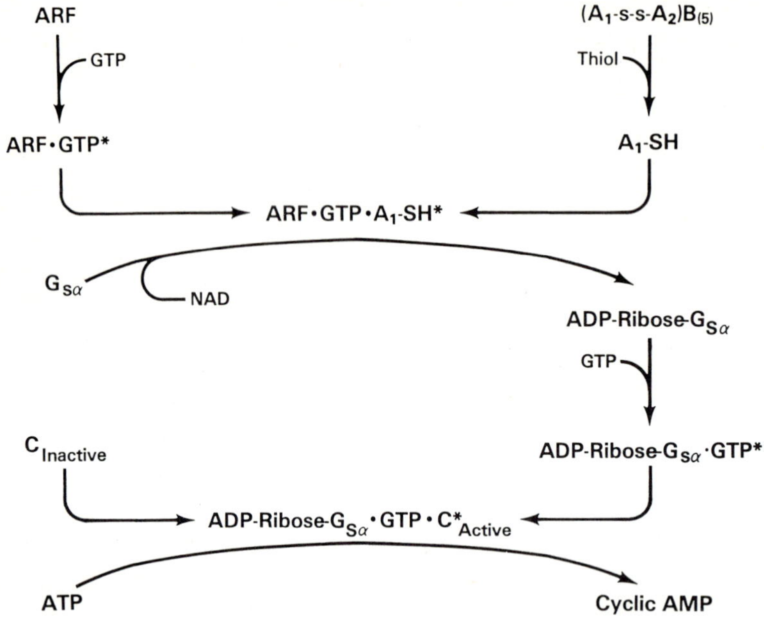

Fig. 1. Proposed G protein cascade for activation of adenylyl cyclase by cholera toxin. Holotoxin is represented as $(A_1\text{-}S\text{-}S\text{-}A_2)B_{(5)}$. ARF·GTP interacts with thiol-activated toxin $(A_1\text{-}SH)$ and stimulates the ADP-ribosyltransferase activity of A_1-SH. ARF-stimulated A_1-SH ADP-ribosylates $G_{s\alpha}$, which binds GTP, becomes constitutively active, and subsequently activates the catalytic subunit of adenylyl cyclase (*C*)

of $G_{s\alpha}$, $G_{t\beta}$, and sARFII was enhanced by DMPC/cholate, whereas ADP-ribosylation of agmatine and auto-ADP-ribosylation of the toxin A1 protein were reduced (TSAI et al. 1988). The sARF-stimulated ADP-ribosylation of other proteins such as phosphorylase b, bovine serum albumin, and α-lactalbumin was not affected by DMPC/cholate (TSAI et al. 1988).

KAHN and GILMAN (1984a) originally proposed that ARF interacted with $G_{s\alpha}$·GTP, thereby improving the ability of $G_{s\alpha}$ to serve as a toxin substrate. In fact, $G_{s\alpha}$·GDP is the toxin substrate; GTPγS (guanosine 5′-*O*-[γ-thio]triphosphate) activation of $G_{s\alpha}$ completely inhibited toxin-catalyzed ADP-ribosylation of $G_{s\alpha}$ and the presence of $\beta\gamma$ subunits did not affect the reaction (KAHN and GILMAN, 1984b). After ARF was shown to be a guanine nucleotide-binding protein, the model was modified to postulate that ARF·GTP interacted with $G_{s\alpha}$ (KAHN and GILMAN 1986). Given that ARF is a guanine nucleotide-binding protein and that ARF·GTP stimulates all of the ADP-ribosyltransferase activities and the NAD glycohydrolase activity of cholera toxin (TSAI et al. 1987, 1988), the guanine nucleotide-binding protein cascade outlined in Fig. 1 for the activation of adenylyl cyclase by ARF-stimulated toxin seems plausible (BOBAK et al. 1990b; MOSS and VAUGHAN 1990; TSAI et al. 1988; VAUGHAN et al. 1989). In

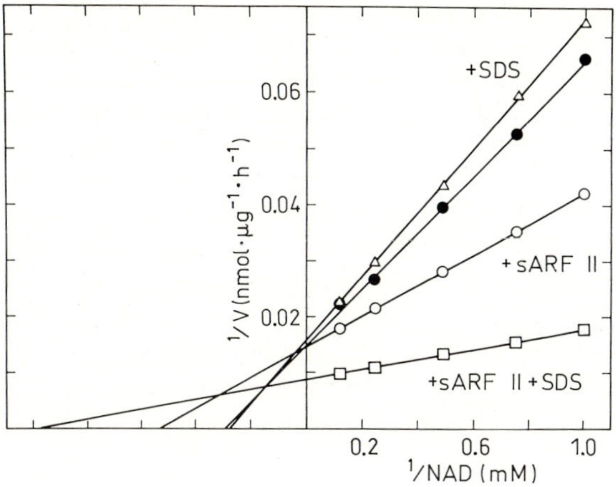

Fig. 2. Lineweaver-Burk analysis of the effect of SDS and sARFII on the cholera toxin-catalyzed NAD: agmatine ADP-ribosyltransferase reaction. ●, no additions; △, SDS; ○, sARFII; □, SDS+sARFII. (Data from NODA et al. 1990)

this model, ARF binds GTP forming the active ARF·GTP complex, which subsequently interacts with the thiol-activated cholera toxin A1 protein, and enhances its enzymatic activities. In the presence of NAD, $G_{s\alpha}$ GDP is ADP-ribosylated by ARF-stimulated toxin and, as described in Sect. 1 of this chapter, ADP-ribosylated $G_{s\alpha}$ binds GTP and subsequently activates adenylyl cyclase.

Support for this model comes from studies that focus on the effects of sARFII on the kinetics of the NAD: agmatine ADP-ribosyltransferase reaction (NODA et al. 1990). In the presence of GTP or a nonhydrolyzable GTP analogue, sARFII stimulated the toxin-catalyzed ADP-ribosylation of agmatine, a simple guanidino compound (NODA et al. 1990; TSAI et al. 1988). The effect of sARFII on the NAD: agmatine ADP-ribosyltransferase activity was enhanced by SDS in a concentration-dependent manner, with 0.003% producing maximal activity; higher concentrations of SDS inhibited both ARF-stimulated and basal activities (NODA et al. 1990). Figure 2 shows a Lineweaver–Burk analysis of the effects of SDS and sARFII on the NAD: agmatine ADP-ribosyltransferase reaction with respect to NAD as substrate. In the absence of SDS, sARFII enhanced the transferase activity by decreasing the K_m for both NAD and agmatine without affecting the V_{max}, whereas, in the presence of SDS, the K_m for each substrate was decreased further and the V_{max} was increased (Fig. 2; NODA et al. 1990). The effect of sARFII was to relieve the negative cooperative effects in the toxin-catalyzed reaction. The effects of ARF were enhanced by SDS, which had minimal effect in the absence of ARF (Fig. 2; NODA et al. 1990).

Over a limited concentration range, cholate (0.1%–0.3%) enhanced sARFII-stimulated NAD: agmatine ADP-ribosyltransferase activity, whereas

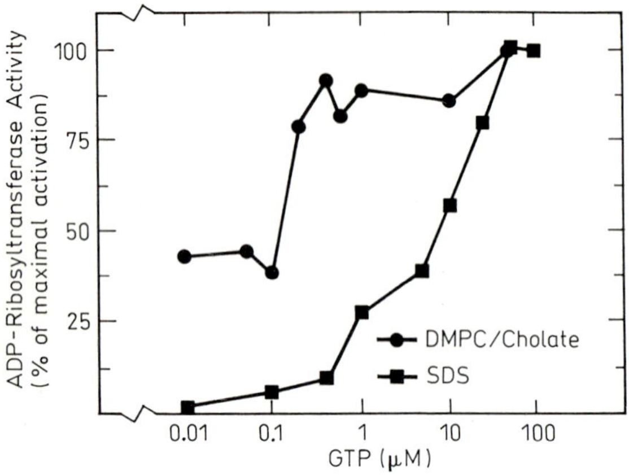

Fig. 3. Effects of SDS or DMPC/cholate on GTP-dependent sARFII-activation of cholera toxin. ■, 0.003% SDS; ● 3m*M* DMPC/0.2% sodium cholate. (Data from NODA et al. in press, see also Moss et al. 1991)

Triton X-100 or CHAPS (3-[(3-cholamidopropyl)-dimethyl-ammonio]-1-propanesultonate) decreased it (NODA et al. 1990). The effect of 0.003% SDS or 3m*M* DMPC/0.2% sodium cholate on GTP activation of sARFII assessed in the NAD: agmatine ADP-ribosyltransferase reaction is shown in Fig. 3 (MOSS et al. 1991; NODA et al., in press). The half maximal effective concentration of GTP in the presence of DMPC/cholate ($K_a \sim 0.2\,\mu M$) is more than an order of magnitude less than that in the absence of detergent or in the presence of SDS ($K_a \sim 9\,\mu M$). These data are consistent with the results of GTP-binding studies in which high affinity binding of GTP ($K_D \sim 70\,nM$) to sARFII was only observed in the presence of DMPC/cholate (BOBAK et al. 1990a).

Binding of GTP to sARFII in the presence of 3m*M* DMPC/0.2% cholate was inhibited at high ionic strength (400 m*M* NaCl) (BOBAK et al. 1990a), whereas mARF required 0.8*M* NaCl for optimal GTPγS binding in the presence of 3m*M* DMPC/0.1% cholate (KAHN and GILMAN 1986). GTP and GDP competed with GTPγS for binding to mARF with apparent dissociation constants of ~90 and ~40 n*M*, respectively, indicating that ARF bound GDP more tightly than GTP (KAHN and GILMAN 1986). High ionic strength also inhibited the binding of guanine nucleotides to a bacterially expressed recombinant ARF (WEISS et al. 1989). Binding of guanine nucleotides to recombinant ARF1 (see discussion below and Fig. 4) was dependent on magnesium concentration (WEISS et al. 1989). In the absence of magnesium, only GDP was bound; at magnesium concentrations of ~10 n*M*, GDP bound to recombinant ARF1 with an apparent affinity ($K_D \sim 1.9\,nM$) ~25-fold greater than that of GTP or GTPγS. Recombinant ARF1 bound all three nucleotides with relatively equal affinities at millimolar concentrations of magnesium (WEISS et al. 1989).

Detergent and phospholipid modified the binding of GTP by ARF as well as the interaction of ARF·GTP with cholera toxin. A fraction of sARFII apparently

```
                  10        20        30        40        50        60
hARF1     MGNIFANLFKGLFGKKEMRILMVGLDAAGKTTILYKLKLGEIVTTIPTIGFNVETVEYKNI
hARF3     *****G**L*S*I************************************************
bARF2     ***V*EK***S**************************************************
hARF4     **LTISS**SR*****Q********************************************
hARF5     **LTVSA**SRI****Q********************************************
hARF6     **KVLSK----I**N*******L*****************QS******V*******T***V
yARF      **LFASK**SN***N***********G*****V********VI*************Q****

                 70        80        90       100       110       120
hARF1     SFTVWDVGGQDKIRPLWRHYFQNTQGLIFVVDSNDRERVNEAREELMRMLAEDELRDAVLL
hARF3     *************************************************************
bARF2     **********************************************T**************
hARF4     C**********R*****K********************IQ*VAD**QK**LV*********
hARF5     C**************************************Q*SAD**QK**Q**********
hARF6     K*N*****************YTG*********CA**D*ID***Q**H*IINDR*M***II*
yARF      ***********R**S*****YR**E*V*********S*IG****VMQ***N*****N*AW*

                130       140       150       160       170       180
hARF1     VFANKQDLPNAMNAAEITDKLGLHSLRHRNWYIQATCATSGDGLYEGLDWLSNQLRNQK
hARF3     ***************************************************A***K*K*
bARF2     **V************************Q***************************K***
hARF4     L***********AIS*M******Q***N*T**V******Q*T***********E*-SKR
hARF5     *******M****PVS*L******QH**S*T**V******Q*T***D******HE*-SKR
hARF6     I********D**KPH**QE****TRI*D****V*PS************T**TSNYKS--
yARF      *********E**S*****E******I*N*P*F*********E******E****S*K*ST
```

Fig. 4. Comparison of ARF-deduced amino acid sequences. Amino acid sequences of human ARFs (hARFs) 1, 3, 4, 5 and 6 (Bobak et al. 1989; Monaco et al. 1990; Tsuchiya et al. 1991), bovine ARF (bARF)2 (Price et al. 1988) and yeast ARF1 (yARF) (Sewell and Kahn 1988), were aligned using CLUSTAL (Higgins and Sharp 1989) as described in Tsuchiya et al. (1991). Amino acid identity with hARF1 is indicated by an *asterisk*; gaps, introduced for optimal alignment, are noted by *hyphens*

complexed and copurified with the toxin A1 protein in the presence of SDS and GTPγS, but not GDPβS (guanosine 5′-*O*-[2-thiodiphosphate]) (Tsai et al. 1991a). No ARF-toxin A1 complex was detected in the presence of DMPC/cholate and GTPγS. The toxin A1 protein complexed with sARFII demonstrated enhanced auto-ADP-ribosyltransferase activity relative to that of the monomeric A1 protein. A small amount of aggregated ARF, with a substrate specificity different from that of monomeric ARF, was formed in the presence of GTPγS alone. Thus, it appears that ARF can complex with itself and/or with the toxin A1 protein under conditions that are GTP-dependent and influenced by phospholipid and detergents. A result of these interactions may be to alter substrate specificity of the toxin. Cholera toxin A1 subunit immobilized on avidin agarose through a biotinylated cysteine near the carboxy terminus was able to catalyze all of the toxin ADP-ribosyltransferase reactions albeit at much reduced rates (Noda et al. 1989). sARFII stimulation of NAD: agmatine and NAD: $G_{s\alpha}$ ADP-ribosyltransferase activities was also apparent but greatly reduced. It was concluded that the cysteine near the carboxy terminus of the toxin A1 subunit is not required for cholera toxin ADP-ribosyltransferase activity or for sARFII regulation. Modification and immobilization of the toxin through this cysteine may, however, limit access to substrate and activator (Noda et al. 1989).

2.2 Molecular and Structural Characterization of ARFs

Six different molecular forms of mammalian *ARF*s and two yeast *ARF* (*yARF*) genes have been cloned and sequenced (Bobak et al. 1989; Monaco et al. 1990; Peng et al. 1989; Price et al. 1988; Sewell and Kahn 1988; Stearns et al. 1990b; Tsuchiya et al. 1991). The mammalian ARFs have been numbered from 1 to 6 based on the order in which they were reported and their relationships to other known ARF sequences (Bobak et al. 1990b). Comparisons of the amino acid sequences of the various forms of ARF (Fig. 4) with sARFII peptide sequence data indicate that sARFII could be ARF1, or ARF3, or both (Bobak et al. 1989). The identity of mARF is unclear; ambiguities in the peptide sequence of mARF make assignment impossible (Sewell and Kahn 1988; Kahn et al. 1988).

ARF2 was cloned from a bovine retinal cDNA library (Price et al. 1988); *ARF1* was cloned from both human and bovine sources (Bobak et al. 1989; Peng et al. 1989; Sewell and Kahn 1988). All of the remaining mammalian *ARF*s (numbers 3–6) were cloned from human cDNA libraries and/or amplified by use of the polymerase chain reaction (PCR) (Bobak et al. 1989; Monaco et al. 1990; Tsuchiya et al. 1991). Deduced amino acid sequences of bovine *ARF1* (*bARF1*) and human *ARF1* (*hARF1*) are 100% identical (Table 2), and those of *hARF6* and a processed chicken pseudogene (*CPS1*) are 99% identical (Table 2), indicating a high degree of conservation across species (Alsip and Konkel 1986; Bobak et al. 1989; Monaco et al. 1990; Sewell and Kahn 1988; Tsuchiya et al. 1991). No human form of *ARF2* has been found either by directly screening a human cDNA library at low stringency (Tsuchiya et al. 1991), PCR amplification of human placental DNA (Monaco et al. 1990), or Northern blot analysis with *bARF2*-specific oligonucleotide probes (Tsuchiya et al. 1989), indicating that *ARF2* may not be well conserved across species.

Deduced amino acid sequences of *hARF*s 1, 3, 4, 5 and 6, *bARF2*, and *yARF1* are shown in Fig. 4[1] (Tsuchiya et al. 1991). *ARF*s*1–3*, *ARF*s*4* and 5, and *ARF6* encode proteins consisting of 181, 180, and 175 amino acids, respectively; all have predicted molecular masses of ~20 kDa (Bobak et al. 1989; Monaco et al. 1990; Peng et al. 1989; Price et al. 1988; Sewell and Kahn 1988; Tsuchiya et al. 1991). There are 181 amino acids in the deduced amino acid sequence of *yARF1* (Sewell and Kahn 1988). As shown in Table 2 and Fig. 4, a high degree of amino acid and nucleotide sequence identity exists among all of the ARF species. In the guanine nucleotide-binding and GTP hydrolysis domains, ARFs share homology with both the α subunits of heterotrimeric G proteins and the small GTP-binding proteins, such as Ras (Bobak et al. 1990b; Price et al. 1990).

Consensus sequences for GTP hydrolysis (Gly-Xaa-Xaa-Xaa-Xaa-Gly-Lys; Asp-Xaa-Xaa-Gly-Gln) and guanine nucleotide binding (Asn-Lys-Xaa-Asp) are found in G protein α subunits, Ras and Ras-like proteins, and all of the ARFs

[1] The nucleotide and deduced amino sequences of the *yARF2* gene were published after completion of this manuscript (Stearns et al. 1990b). Like yARF1, yARF2 consists of 181 amino acids and contains the consensus sequences for guanine nucleotide binding and GTP hydrolysis found in all ARFs, in the same positions as in yARF1

Table 2. Comparison of nucleotide and deduced amino acid sequences of ADP-ribosylation factors

	hARF1	bARF1	bARF2	hARF3	hARF4	hARF5	hARF6	CPS1	yARF
hARF1	—	100	96	96	80	80	68	67	77
bARF1	91	—	96	96	80	80	68	67	77
bARF2	79	80	—	95	80	80	69	68	77
hARF3	84	84	80	—	79	79	68	68	76
hARF4	67	68	68	71	—	90	64	64	72
hARF5	75	73	71	73	77	—	64	64	69
hARF6	68	69	64	66	60	65	—	99	65
CPS1	69	68	63	68	60	65	89	—	65
yARF	64	66	66	65	67	64	60	59	—

Percentage identity of the deduced amino acid sequences of human ARFs (hARFs), 1, 3–6 (Bobak et al. 1989; Monaco et al. 1990; Tsuchiya et al. 1991), bovine ARFs (bARFs) 1 and 2 (Price et al. 1988; Sewell and Kahn 1988), the chicken pseudogene (CPS1) (Alsip and Konkel 1986) and yeast ARF1 (yARF) (Sewell and Kahn 1988) is indicated above the diagonal, and percentage identity of nucleotide sequences (coding regions) is below the diagonal as described in Tsuchiya et al. (1991)

(Price et al. 1990). In ARFs 1–5 and yARF1 these regions are at amino acid positions 24–30, 67–71, and 126–129, respectively (Fig. 4); in ARF6 these correspond to positions 20–26, 63–67, and 122–125, respectively (Fig. 4). The sequence Cys-Ala-Thr, at positions 159–161 in ARFs 1–5 and yARF1 and 155–157 in ARF6 (Fig. 4), is also believed to be involved in guanine nucleotide binding. This sequence is present in most G protein α subunits but is different in Ras and Ras-related small GTP-binding proteins (Price et al. 1990). In this regard, ARF appears more closely related to G protein α subunits than to Ras. Nevertheless, based on size, sequence similarities, and relatedness to one another, the ARFs constitute a distinct family of small GTP-binding proteins.

The active form of ARF is the GTP-liganded species. Although ARF isolated from membranes contains stoichiometric amounts of GDP (Kahn and Gilman 1986), no ARF GTPase activity has been detected (Kahn and Gilman 1986; Weiss et al. 1989). In Ras, replacement of Gly-12 with any amino acid except proline results in reduced GTPase activity (Gibbs et al. 1984; McGrath et al. 1984; Sweet et al. 1984). Glycine occurs in the corresponding position in G protein α subunits, but in ARF the corresponding amino acid is Asp-26 (Price et al. 1990). This difference may account, at least in part, for the observed lack of ARF GTPase activity.

The amino termini of purified mARF and sARFII were blocked to Edman degradation (Kahn et al. 1988; Price et al. 1988), and the blocking group in mARF was identified as myristoylglycine (Kahn et al. 1988). In all of the ARF deduced amino acid sequences (Fig. 4 and Stearns et al. 1990b) a glycine is present next to the initiating methionine, removal of which results in a protein with an amino-terminal glycine that may be modified by myristoyl-CoA:protein *N*-myristoyl transferase. Mammalian ARFs 1, 4, and 5, yARF1 (Fig. 4), and yARF2 (Stearns et al. 1990b) each contain a Ser, Thr, or Ala as the fifth amino acid downstream from the amino-terminal glycine which is believed to be part of the recognition site for the transferase (Towler et al. 1987). ARFs 2 and 3 have a glutamate and a glycine, respectively, at this position. Nevertheless, recombinant ARF2 can be myristylated (Kunz et al. 1990). Lack of myristate on bacterially expressed recombinant ARF1 did not affect its guanine nucleotide-binding properties or its ability to stimulate toxin-catalyzed ADP-ribosylation of $G_{s\alpha}$ (Weiss et al. 1989). However, the activity of recombinant ARF1 was much more sensitive to high ionic strength than was that of mARF purified from bovine brain. It is unclear whether myristylation affects salt sensitivity.

The family of mammalian ARFs can be divided into three major classes based on molecular size and amino acid identity. Class I includes ARFs 1–3. Each consists of 181 amino acids with differences in deduced amino acid sequence primarily near the amino and carboxy termini (Fig. 4). Class II includes ARFs 4 and 5, each with 180 amino acids and differences scattered throughout the sequences. Nevertheless, they are more similar to each other than to class I ARFs. Class III consists of ARF6 with 175 amino acids. It diverges from ARFs 1–5 throughout its sequence, with significantly more differences noted near the amino terminus and in the carboxy half of the protein. The results of

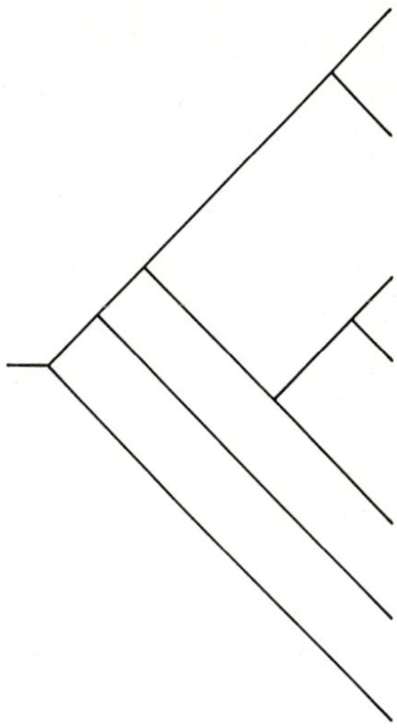

Fig. 5. Phylogenetic analysis of ARF cDNA coding regions. Nucleotide sequences of the coding regions of *hARFs 1–6*, *bARF2*, and *yARF* (*yARF1*) were aligned as described in TSUCHIYA et al. (1991). An evolutionary tree was constructed using the DNADIST and KITSCH programs of the PHYLIP phylogenetic software package. Branch lengths do not correlate with evolutionary time

phylogenetic analysis of the ARFs (Fig. 5) are consistent with the conclusion that the six mammalian ARFs fall into three separate classes, and that ARFs 1–3 and ARFs 4 and 5 are more closely related to each other than they are to ARFs outside their groups. In this analysis, yARF1 also falls into a distinct class. Despite the differences among the ARFs, they clearly represent a family of proteins distinct from other ~20-kDa guanine nucleotide-binding proteins (e.g., Ras, Rho, Ral).

2.3 Distribution of ARF mRNAs and Proteins

Each ARF appears to be the product of separate genes. As summarized in Fig. 6, ARF-specific oligonucleotide probes hybridized to brain poly(A)$^+$ RNA, producing distinct mRNA patterns. ARF1-specific oligonucleotides hybridized to a single mRNA species of 1.7–2.1 kb from bovine, human, rat, mouse, and rabbit (BOBAK et al. 1989; KAHN and SEWELL 1988; TSUCHIYA et al. 1989). In all species examined, ARF4-specific oligonucleotides hybridized to a ~1.8-kb mRNA, whereas ARF5-specific probes hybridized to a ~1.3-kb mRNA (MONACO et al. 1990; TSUCHIYA et al. 1991). ARF3 and ARF6 mRNAs are also widespread and appear to be present in multiple forms. ARF3-specific oligonucleotides hybridized to two bands of 3.7–3.8 and 1.2–1.3 kb (BOBAK et al. 1989), whereas ARF6-specific probes hybridized to 4.2- and 1.8-kb bands (TSUCHIYA et al. 1991). In contrast, ARF2 mRNA was not detected in all species. A single ARF2-specific mRNA band of 2.1–2.6 kb was observed in brain poly(A)$^+$ RNA from bovine, rat, and mouse, but not from human or monkey (PRICE et al. 1988; TSUCHIYA

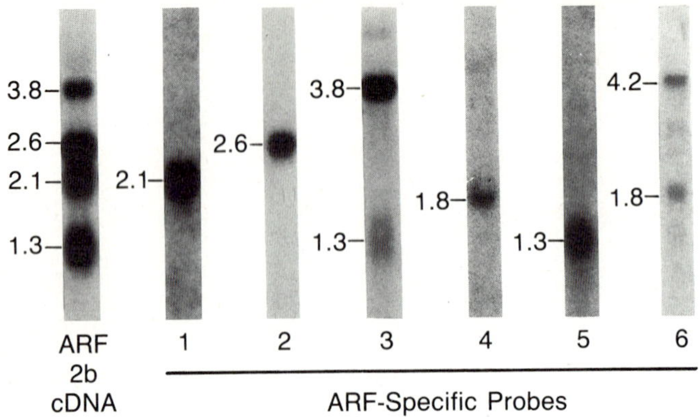

Fig. 6. Size distribution and patterns of ARF-specific mRNAs. Rat brain poly(A)$^+$ RNA was hybridized with ARF-specific oligonucleotide probes: 1, complementary to bases 4–51 of *hARF1* BOBAK et al. 1989); 2, complementary to bases 267–314 of *bARF2* (PRICE et al. 1988); 3, complementary to bases 4–51 of *hARF3* (BOBAK et al. 1989); 4, complementary to bases -5 to 30 of *hARF4* (MONACO et al. 1989); 5, complementary to bases 350–381 of *hARF5*; and 6, complementary to bases 825–854 of *hARF6* (TSUCHIYA et al. 1991). The ARF2b cDNA probe is the 592-bp *Eco*RI-*Pvu*II fragment containing the *bARF2* coding region (PRICE et al. 1988). Labeling and hybridization conditions are described in TSUCHIYA et al. (1989, 1991)

et al. 1989; STEVENS et al., unpublished observations). Oligonucleotide probes complementary to the 3'- and 5'- untranslated regions of *hARF1* and *bARF2* did not hybridize with mRNA across species, consistent with the view that the ARF coding regions are more highly conserved than the untranslated regions (BOBAK et al. 1989; TSUCHIYA et al. 1989).

mRNAs corresponding to ARFs 1–6 were detected in numerous tissues, including brain, lung, heart, kidney, spleen, and retina (TSUCHIYA et al. 1989, 1991). In bovine tissues ARF2 mRNA was primarily in brain, lung, and kidney with only traces in liver, whereas ARF1 mRNA was more widespread with the highest concentrations in brain and lung (TSUCHIYA et al. 1989). ARF-immunoreactive material was primarily cytosolic and most abundant in neural tissues (KAHN et al. 1988; TSAI et al. 1991b). The sARF-immunoreactive proteins ran as a doublet on SDS-polyacrylamide gels (Fig. 7); the upper band (sARFII) was more intense in brain, whereas the lower band (sARFI) predominated in peripheral tissues (TSAI et al. 1991b). ARF immunoreactivity was observed in every eukaryotic species studied, including human, bovine, rat, mouse, rabbit, frog, chicken, yeast, and slime mold (Fig. 7; KAHN et al. 1988; TSAI et al. 1991b). On the other hand, it was not detected in *Escherichia coli* (KAHN et al. 1988).

A differential pattern of ARF expression was observed during development of rat brain (TSAI et al. 1991b). Using antiserum prepared against sARFII, which recognizes both sARFI and sARFII, developmental changes in immunoreactive sARFI and sARFII were followed. At 2 days postnatally, levels of immunoreactive sARFI and sARFII were approximately equal, whereas by 10 days postnatally

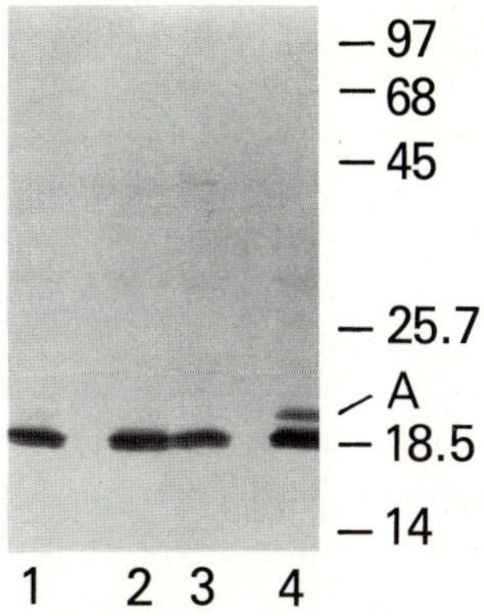

Fig. 7. Species distribution of immunoreactive ARF. Proteins from bovine (*lane 1*), rat (*lane 2*), frog (*lane 3*), and chicken (*lane 4*) brain cytosol were separated by electrophoresis in an 18% SDS-polyacrylamide gel, transferred to nitrocellulose paper, and reacted with anti-sARFII antibodies. Standard proteins are phosphorylase b (97 kDa), bovine serum albumin (68 kDa), ovalbumin (45 kDa), α-chymotrypsinogen (25.7 kDa), β-lactoglobulin (18.5 kDa) and lysozyme (14 kDa). *A* is a chicken-specific ARF-immunoreactive band which is apparently larger than sARFI and sARFII. (Data from TSAI et al. 1991b)

sARFII was the predominant form. These results correlated with increases in ARF3-specific mRNA and decreases in ARF2- and ARF4-specific mRNA between 2 and 27 days postnatally. Levels of ARF1-, ARF5- and ARF6-specific mRNA appeared unchanged over this period. The partial peptide sequence of sARFII is consistent with it being the product of ARF1, or ARF3, or both mRNAs (BOBAK et al. 1989). Based on these data it is tempting to speculate that sARFII is, or includes, the product of the ARF3 gene.

2.4 Physiological Function(s) of ARFs

The physiological function of ARF is unknown. Since there are at least six different forms of mammalian ARF, forming three distinct classes of proteins, more than one function is possible. ARF was first identified by its ability to stimulate cholera toxin activation of adenylyl cyclase and toxin-catalyzed ADP-ribosylation of $G_{s\alpha}$ in vitro. There is no evidence that ARF serves this function in vivo. Another possibility is that ARF regulates the activity of intracellular NAD: arginine ADP-ribosyltransferases. However, despite the fact that ARF stimulates all of the ADP-ribosyltransferase activities of cholera toxin, it has no demonstrable effect on the activities of four purified eukaryotic NAD: arginine ADP-ribosyltransferases (MOSS and STANLEY, unpublished observations).

ARF may play a role in the oocyte maturation process, Microinjection of sARFII into *Xenopus laevis* oocytes inhibited both progesterone- and insulin-stimulated maturation (BAHNSON et al. 1989). Injection of sARFII had no observable effects on unstimulated cells. ARF-induced inhibition was enhanced by GTP and GTPγS, but not GDP; GTPγS was more potent than GTP. It was suggested that ARF may affect the maturation process at a point after the convergence of progesterone- and insulin-dependent pathways. This could be a cAMP-mediated event, since oocyte maturation is stimulated by a decrease in cAMP and inhibited by stimulation of cAMP-dependent protein kinase (MALLER and KREBS 1977). Alternatively, ARF inhibition of oocyte maturation could result from a more general effect on cytoskeletal function or intracellular protein movement.

Vectorial transport of proteins through the Golgi system requires the participation of ~20-kDa GTP-binding proteins (for reviews, see BALCH 1989; HALL 1990; ROTHMAN and ORCI 1990) such as SEC4 (SALMINEN and NOVICK 1987) and YPT1 (SEGEV et al. 1988) which function late (post-Golgi) and early (ER-Golgi) in yeast protein transport stages, respectively. Mutational studies in yeast suggest a role for ARF in the transport process. There are two yeast ARF genes, *yARF1* (yARF, Fig. 6) and *yARF2* (STEARNS et al. 1990b). *yARF1* accounts for ~90% of the total cellular ARF protein and *yARF2* for ~10% (STEARNS et al. 1990b). These two genes encode proteins that are more than 96% identical in amino acid sequences. Deletion of both yARF genes is lethal, whereas deletion of *yARF2* produces a mutant that is indistinguishable from wild type. On the other hand, the *arf1* null mutant that lacks the *yARF1* gene is cold-sensitive, slow-growing, and supersensitive to fluoride ions (STEARNS et al. 1990b). These mutant cells accumulated an intermediate glycosylated form of invertase, not seen in wild-type cells, consistent with the existence of a partial glycosylation defect in the secretory pathway (STEARNS et al. 1990a); a similar defect was observed in mutants of *YPT1* (SALMINEN and NOVICK 1987). However, mutants of *YPT1* and *yARF1* do not complement each other (STEARNS et al. 1990a). Yeast *SEC18* mutants also exhibit a glycosylation defect in the secretory pathway. In *sec18-1* temperature-sensitive mutants, movement of invertase from the ER to the Golgi apparatus is blocked (ESMON et al. 1981). At the nonpermissive temperature, invertase can only be core-glycosylated in these cells (ESMON et al. 1981). Analysis of a temperature-sensitive double mutant defective in *yARF1* at the permissive temperature and in *SEC18* at the nonpermissive temperature indicated that the *yARF1*-dependent stage of the secretory process was a later event than the *SEC18*-dependent stage (STEARNS et al. 1990a).

Immunofluorescence studies, with affinity-purified anti-ARF peptide antibodies prepared against amino acids 25–36 of bARF1, localized ARF predominantly in the stacked Golgi cisternae of NIH3T3 and SW13 human adrenal carcinoma cells (STEARNS et al. 1990a). Immunoelectron microscopic studies localized ARF staining predominantly to *cis* elements of the cytoplasmic face of the Golgi stack (STEARNS et al. 1990a). These data and the yeast mutational studies are consistent with a role for ARF in protein transport through the Golgi system.

3 Effect of ARF on *E. coli* Heat-Labile Enterotoxins

"Traveler's diarrhea" is caused, in part, by strains of *E. coli* that secrete heat-labile (LT) or heat-stable (ST) enterotoxins (for review, see CARPENTER 1980; HOLMGREN and LÖNNROTH 1980; MOSS and VAUGHAN 1988a,b). LT is similar to cholera toxin in structure and in function. It is composed of one A and five B subunits (CLEMENTS et al. 1980; CLEMENTS and FINKELSTEIN 1979; ROBERTSON et al. 1980) and activates adenylyl cyclase via an NAD-dependent mechanism (GILL et al. 1976). Like cholera toxin, LT possesses NAD glycohydrolase as well as NAD: arginine and NAD: protein mono-ADP-ribosyltransferase activities (GILL and RICHARDSON et al. 1980; MOSS and RICHARDSON 1978; MOSS et al. 1979b, 1981). Expression of the latent activities requires activation of the A subunit with dithiothreitol and trypsin generating the active A1 protein (MOSS and RICHARDSON 1978; MOSS et al. 1981).

The LT family includes two major serotypes, LT-I and LT-II, and their subtypes. LT-I is similar to cholera toxin in amino acid sequence, ganglioside binding, and immunoreactivity (MOSS and VAUGHAN 1988a[2]); in contrast to cholera toxin, LT-I may use glycoprotein(s) as well as ganglioside G_{M1} as its

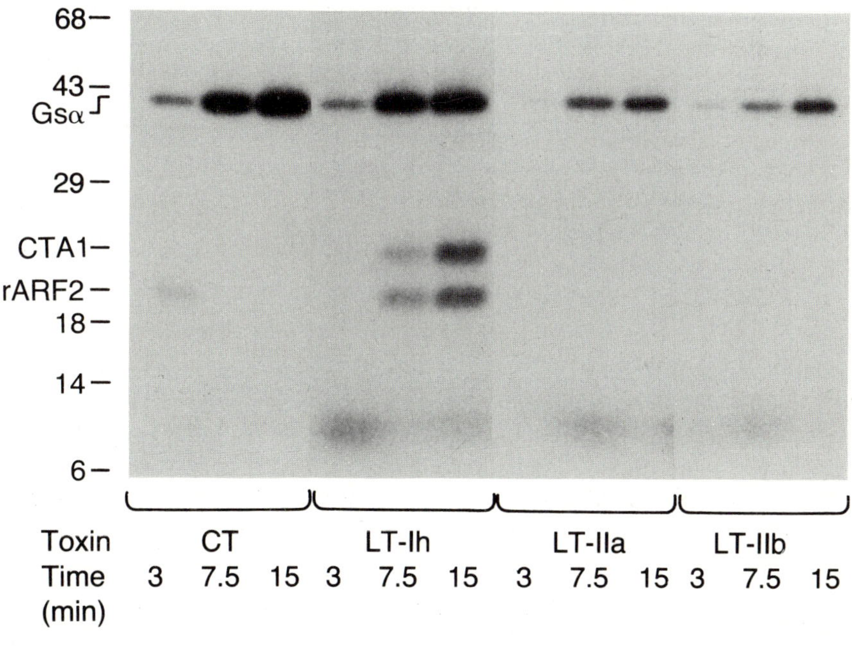

Fig. 8. ADP-ribosylation of $G_{s\alpha}$ by cholera toxin (*CT*) and three *E. coli* heat-labile enterotoxins (LT-Ih, LT-IIa, LT-IIb). G_s was incubated with activated toxin for 3–15 min in the presence of GTP, recombinant ARF2 (*rARF2*), 0.9 m*M* DMPC/0.06% sodium cholate and [^{32}P]NAD. [^{32}P]ADP-ribosylated $G_{s\alpha}$ was assessed after electrophoresis in 14% SDS-polyacrylamide gels. Standard proteins are bovine serum albumin (68 kDa), ovalbumin (43 kDa), carbonic anhydrase (29 kDa), β-lactoglobulin (18 kDa), lysozyme (14 kDa), and bovine trypsin inhibitor (6 kDa). *CTA1* is cholera toxin A1 subunit. (Data from LEE et al. 1991)

---

[2] Unless stated otherwise, it appears that the heat-labile enterotoxin discussed in the references cited in this article is LT-I

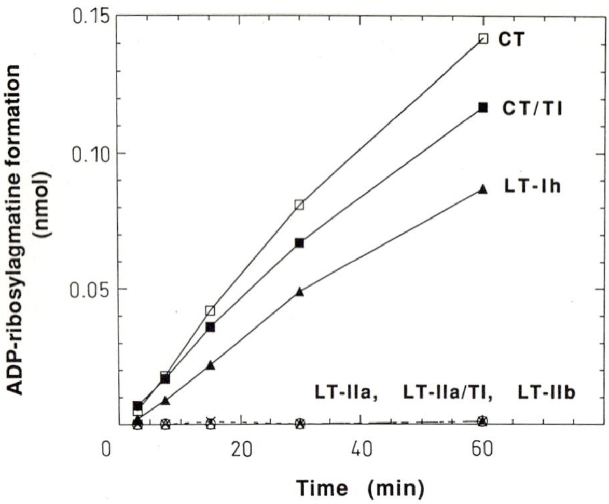

Fig. 9. ARF-stimulated toxin-catalyzed ADP-ribosylagmatine formation. The NAD: agmatine ADP-ribosyltransferase activities of cholera toxin (*CT*) and the heat-labile enterotoxins (LT-Ih, LT-IIa, LT-IIb) were assayed at various times in the presence of GTP, recombinant ARF2, 0.9 m*M* DMPC/0.06% sodium cholate, and trypsin. Soybean trypsin inhibitor (*TI*) was added at zero time to the CT and LT-IIa reactions as indicated. ADP-ribosylagmatine formation was assayed for the different toxins: cholera toxin (-□-), cholera toxin + soybean trypsin inhibitor (-■-), LT-Ih (-▲-), LT-IIa (-○-), LT-IIa + soybean trypsin inhibitor, LT-IIb (-×-). (Data from LEE et al. 1991)

cellular receptor (HOLMGREN 1973; HOLMGREN et al. 1982, 1985; MOSS et al. 1979a, 1981; PIERCE 1973). The LT-II family differs from LT-I in amino acid sequence, ganglioside binding, and immunoreactivity (CHANG et al. 1987; HOLMES et al. 1986; PICKETT et al. 1986). Despite these differences, all of the toxins appear to activate adenylyl cyclase via a mechanism involving ADP-ribosylation (CHANG et al. 1987; FINKELSTEIN 1973; KELLY 1986; MOSS and VAUGHAN 1988a). Cholera toxin, LT-Ih, LT-IIa, and LT-IIb ADP-ribosylated the α subunit of purified G_s (Fig. 8; LEE et al. 1991). In each instance, ARF, GTP, and DMPC/cholate were required for optimal acitvity (LEE et al. 1991). As observed with cholera toxin, ARF·GTP stimulated the NAD: agmatine ADP-ribosyltransferase activities of LT-Ih, LT-IIa, and LT-IIb; activation by ARF·GTP was enhanced by SDS. ARF·GTP also stimulated the auto-ADP-ribosylation of each toxin (LEE et al.1991). LT-IIa and LT-IIb utilized $G_{s\alpha}$ (Fig. 8) at rates similar to those of cholera toxin and LT-Ih; in contrast, agmatine was utilized by LT-IIa and LT-IIb at rates much less than those observed with LT-Ih or cholera toxin (Figs. 8 and 9; LEE et al. 1991). Although the genes for the A subunits of cholera toxin, LT-I and LT-IIs exhibit some differences (MOSS and VAUGHAN 1988a; PICKETT and HOLMES, in press; PICKETT et al. 1986, 1987, 1989), the mechanism of action and the allosteric activation site utilized by ARF have been conserved.

4 Conclusions

Understanding the role of G proteins in regulating the adenylyl cyclase system was facilitated, in part, by elucidating the mechanism of cholera toxin action. The ADP-ribosyltransferase activity of cholera toxin was a valuable tool in these endeavors and even now continues to be important in studies that focus on the functional domains of G proteins (BOURNE et al. 1989; FREISSMUTH and GILMAN 1989; LANDIS et al. 1989). It led also to the discovery of a family of soluble and membrane ARFs whose physiological function(s) are not yet understood. At present, ARFs are characterized functionally by their ability to bind guanine nucleotides and stimulate the ADP-ribosyltransferase activities of cholera toxin in vitro (Sect. 2).

$G_{s\alpha}$ is the only well-established physiological cholera toxin substrate. In HL-60 cell membranes, the 40-kDa inhibitory G protein, $G_{i\alpha 2}$ is ADP-ribosylated by cholera toxin only when it is coupled to receptor (IIRI et al. 1989). It is not clear what effect cholera toxin-catalyzed ADP-ribosylation of $G_{i\alpha 2}$ has on these cells. Toxin-catalyzed ADP-ribosylation of numerous membrane and cytosolic proteins occurs in vitro (GILL and COBURN 1987; COOPER et al. 1981; HAWKINS and BROWNING 1982; TSAI et al. 1987, 1988; WATKINS et al. 1980). cAMP-independent toxin effects on receptor-mediated Ca^{2+} mobilization and phosphoinositide metabolism have been observed in several types of cells (IMBODEN et al. 1986; LO and HUGHES 1987; NARASIMHAN et al. 1988; MCCLOSKEY 1988; PIKE and EAKES 1987). Cholera toxin also inhibited chemotaxis by a cAMP-independent mechanism in RAW 264 mouse macrophage cells (AKSAMIT et al. 1985). These observations may reflect the multiple functions of $G_{s\alpha}$, which can regulate Ca^{2+} channels (MATTERA et al. 1989; YATANI et al. 1988) as well as adenylyl cyclase, and/or the effect(s) of toxin binding or toxin-catalyzed ADP-ribosylation of other proteins.

Understanding the structure and properties of cholera toxin has led to a better understanding of similar toxins, such as the *E. coli* heat-labile enterotoxins (Sect. 3). Its ADP-ribosyltransferase activity has been a valuable tool in understanding the adenylyl cyclase system (Sect. 1) and has led to the discovery of ARFs (Sect. 2). Perhaps, it will also be of value in elucidating the mechanisms of chemotaxis, receptor-mediated Ca^{2+} mobilization, and regulation of phosphoinositide metabolism.

Acknowledgement. We thank Ms. Carol Kosh for expert secretarial assistance.

References

Abood ME, Hurley JB, Pappone M-C, Bourne HR, Stryer L (1982) Functional homology between signal-coupling proteins. J Biol Chem 257: 10540–10543

Aksamit RR, Backlund PS Jr, Cantoni GL (1985) Cholera toxin inhibits chemotaxis by a cAMP-independent mechanism. Proc Natl Acad Sci USA 82: 7475–7479

Alsip GR, Konkel DA (1986) A processed chicken pseudogene (CPS1) related to the *ras* oncogene superfamily. Nucleic Acids Res 14: 2123–2138

Bahnson TD, Tsai S-C, Adamik R, Moss J, Vaughan M (1989) Microinjection of a 19-kDa guanine nucleotide-binding protein inhibits maturation of *Xenopus* oocytes. J Biol Chem 264: 14824–14828

Balch WE (1989) Biochemistry of interorganelle transport. J Biol Chem 264: 16965–16968

Birnbaumer L, Codina J, Mattera R, Yatani A, Scherer N, Toro M-J, Brown AM (1987) Signal transduction by G proteins. Kidney Int [Suppl 23] 32: S14–S37

Birnbaumer L, Mattera R, Yatani A, Codina J, van Dongen AMJ, Brown AM (1990) Recent advances in the understanding of multiple roles of G proteins in coupling of receptors to ionic channels and other effectors. In: Moss J, Vaughan M (eds) ADP-ribosylating toxins and G proteins: insights into signal transduction. American Society for Microbiology, Washington

Bobak DA, Nightingale MS, Murtagh JJ, Price SR, Moss J, Vaughan M (1989) Molecular cloning, characterization, and expression of human ADP-ribosylation factors: two guanine nucleotide-dependent activators of cholera toxin. Proc Natl Acad Sci USA 86: 6101–6105

Bobak DA, Bliziotes MM, Noda M, Tsai S-C, Adamik R, Moss J (1990a) Mechanism of activation of cholera toxin by ADP-ribosylation factor (ARF): both low- and high-affinity interactions of ARF with guanine nucleotides promote toxin activation. Biochemistry 29: 855–861

Bobak DA, Tsai S-C, Moss, J, Vaughan M (1990b) Enhancement of cholera toxin ADP-ribosyltransferase activity by guanine nucleotide-dependent ADP-ribosylation factors. In: Moss J, Vaughan M (eds) ADP-ribosylating toxins and G proteins: insights into signal transduction. American Society for Microbiology, Washington

Bourne HR, Landis CA, Masters SB (1989) Hydrolysis of GTP by the α-chain of G_s and other GTP binding proteins. Proteins 6: 222–230

Bray P, Carter A, Simons C, Guo V, Puckett C, Kamholz J, Spiegel A, Nirenberg M (1986) Human cDNA clones for four species of $G_{s\alpha}$ signal transduction protein. Proc Natl Acad Sci USA 83: 8893–8897

Burns DL, Moss J, Vaughan M (1982) Choleragen-stimulated release of guanyl nucleotides from turkey erythrocyte membranes. J Biol Chem 257: 32–34

Burns DL, Moss J, Vaughan M (1983) Release of guanyl nucleotides from the regulatory subunit of adenylate cyclase. J Biol Chem 258: 1116–1120

Carpenter CCJ (1980) Clinical and pathophysiologic features of diarrhea caused by *Vibrio cholerae* and *Escherichia coli*. In: Field M, Fordtran JS, Schultz SG (eds) Secretory diarrhea. American Physiological Society, Bethesda

Casey PJ, Gilman AG (1988) G protein involvement in receptor-effector coupling. J Biol Chem 263: 2577–2580

Cassel D, Pfeuffer T (1978) Mechanism of cholera toxin action: covalent modification of the guanyl nucleotide-binding protein of the adenylate cyclase system. Proc Natl Acad Sci USA 75: 2669–2673

Cassel D, Selinger Z (1977) Mechanism of adenylate cyclase activation by cholera toxin: inhibition of GTP hydrolysis at the regulatory site. Proc Natl Acad Sci USA 74: 3307–3311

Chang F-H, Bourne HR (1989) Cholera toxin induces cAMP-independent degradation of G_s. J Biol Chem 264: 5352–5357

Chang PP, Fishman PH, Ohtomo N, Moss J (1983) Degradation of choleragen bound to cultured human fibroblasts and mouse neuroblastoma cells. J Biol Chem 258: 426–430

Chang PP, Moss J, Twiddy EM, Holmes RK (1987) Type II heat-labile enterotoxin of *Escherichia coli* activates adenylate cyclase in human fibroblasts by ADP-ribosylation. Infect Immun 55: 1854–1858

Clements JD, Finkelstein RA (1979) Isolation and characterization of homogenous heat-labile enterotoxins with high specific activity from *Escherichia coli* cultures. Infect Immun 24: 760–769

Clements JD, Yancey RJ, Finkelstein RA (1980) Properties of homogenous heat-labile enterotoxin from *Escherichia coli*. Infect Immun 29: 91–97

Cooper DMF, Jagus R, Somers RL, Rodbell M (1981) Cholera toxin modifies diverse GTP-modulated regulatory proteins. Biochem Biophys Res Commun 101: 1179–1185

Cuatrecasas P (1973a) Interaction of *Vibrio cholerae* enterotoxin with cell membranes. Biochemistry 12: 3547–3558

Cuatrecasas P (1973b) Gangliosides and membrane receptors for cholera toxin. Biochemistry 12: 3558–3566

Cuatrecasas P (1973c) *Vibrio cholerae* choleragenoid: mechanism of inhibition of cholera toxin action. Biochemistry 12: 3577–3581

Enomoto K, Asakawa T (1982) Partial purification and properties of a cytosolic protein factor required for the activation of rat liver adenylate cyclase by cholera toxin. Biomed Res 3: 122–131

Enomoto K, Gill DM (1979) Requirement for guanosine triphosphate in the activation of adenylate cyclase by cholera toxin. J Supramol Struct 10: 51–60

Enomoto K, Gill DM (1980) Cholera toxin activation of adenylate cyclase. J Biol Chem 255: 1252–1258

Esmon B, Novick P, Schekman R (1981) Compartmentalized assembly of oligosaccharides on exported glycoproteins in yeast. Cell 25: 451–460

Finkelstein RA (1973) Cholera. CRC Crit Rev Microbiol 2: 553–623

Fishman PH, Moss J, Osborne JC Jr (1978) Interaction of choleragen with the oligosaccharide of ganglioside GM_1: evidence for multiple oligosaccharide binding sites. Biochemistry 17: 711–716

Freissmuth M, Gilman AG (1989) Mutations of $G_{s\alpha}$ designed to alter the reactivity of the protein with bacterial toxins. J Biol Chem 264: 21907–21914

Gibbs JB, Sigal IS, Poe M, Scolnick EM (1984) Intrinsic GTPase activity distinguishes normal and oncogenic *ras* p21 molecules. Proc Natl Acad Sci USA 81: 5704–5708

Gill DM (1975) Involvement of nicotinamide adenine dinucleotide in the action of cholera toxin in vitro. Proc Natl Acad Sci USA 72: 2064–2068

Gill DM (1976a) The arrangement of subunits in cholera toxin. Biochemistry 15: 1242–1248

Gill DM (1976b) Multiple roles of erythrocyte supernatant in the activation of adenylate cyclase by *Vibrio cholerae* toxin in vitro. J Infect Dis 133: S55–S63

Gill DM (1977) Mechanism of action of cholera toxin. Adv Cyclic Nucleotide Res 8: 85–118

Gill DM, Coburn J (1987) ADP-ribosylation by cholera toxin: functional analysis of a cellular system that stimulates the enzymic activity of cholera toxin fragment A_1. Biochemistry 26: 6364–6371

Gill DM, King CA (1975) The mechanism of action of cholera toxin in pigeon erythrocyte lysates. J Biol Chem 250: 6424–6432

Gill DM, Meren R (1978) ADP-ribosylation of membrane proteins catalyzed by cholera toxin: basis of the activation of adenylate cyclase. Proc Natl Acad Sci USA 75: 3050–3054

Gill DM, Meren R (1983) A second guanyl nucleotide-binding site associated with adenylate cyclase. J Biol Chem 258: 11908–11914

Gill DM, Rappaport RS (1979) Origin of the enzymatically active A_1 fragment of cholera toxin. J Infect Dis 139: 674–680

Gill DM, Richardson SH (1980) Adenosine diphosphate-ribosylation of adenylate cyclase catalyzed by heat-labile enterotoxin of *Escherichia coli*: comparison with cholera toxin. J Infect Dis 141: 64–70

Gill DM, Woolkalis M (1988) [^{32}P]ADP-ribosylation of proteins catalyzed by cholera toxin and related heat-labile enterotoxins. Methods Enzymol 165: 235–245

Gill DM, Evans DJ Jr, Evans DG (1976) Mechanism of activation of adenylate cyclase in vitro by polymyxin-released, heat-labile enterotoxin of *Escherichia coli*. J Infect Dis 133: S103–S107

Gilman AG (1987) G proteins: transducers of receptor-generated signals. Annu Rev Biochem 56: 615–649

Graves CB, Klaven NB, McDonald JM (1983) Effects of guanine nucleotides on cholera toxin catalyzed ADP-ribosylation in rat adipocyte plasma membranes. Biochemistry 22: 6291–6296

Hall A (1990) The cellular functions of small GTP-binding proteins. Science 249: 635–640

Hawkins DJ, Browning ET (1982) Tubulin adenosine diphosphate ribosylation is catalyzed by cholera toxin. Biochemistry 21: 4474–4479

Higgins DG, Sharp PM (1989) Fast and sensitive multiple sequence alignments on a microcomputer. CABIOS 5: 151–153

Holmes RK, Twiddy EM, Pickett CL (1986) Purification and characterization of type II heat-labile enterotoxin of *Escherichia coli*. Infect Immun 53: 464–473

Holmgren J (1973) Comparison of the tissue receptors for *Vibrio cholerae* and *Escherichia coli* enterotoxins by means of gangliosides and natural cholera toxoid. Infect Immun 8: 851–859

Holmgren J, Lönnroth I (1980) Structure and function of enterotoxins and their receptor. In: Ouchterlony O, Holmgren J (eds) Cholera and related diarrheas. Karger, Basel

Holmgren J, Lönnroth I, Svennerholm L (1973) Tissue receptor for cholera exotoxin: postulated structure from studies with G_{M1} ganglioside and related glycolipids. Infect Immun 8: 208–214

Holmgren J, Månsson J-E, Svennerholm L (1974) Tissue receptor for cholera exotoxin: structural requirements of G_{M1} ganglioside in toxin binding and inactivation. Med Biol 52: 229–233

Holmgren J, Fredman P, Lindblad M, Svennerholm A-M, Svennerholm L (1982) Rabbit intestinal glycoprotein receptor for *Escherichia coli* heat-labile enterotoxin lacking affinity for cholera toxin. Infect Immun 38: 424–433

Holmgren J, Lindblad M, Fredman P, Svennerholm L, Myrvold H (1985) Comparison of receptor for cholera and *Escherichia coli* enterotoxins in human intestine. Gastroenterology 89: 27–35

Iiri T, Tohkin M, Morishima N, Ohoka Y, Ui M, Katada T (1989) Chemotactic peptide receptor-supported ADP-ribosylation of a pertussis toxin substrate GTP-binding protein by cholera toxin in neutrophil-type HL-60 cells. J Biol Chem 264: 21394–21400

Imboden JB, Shoback DM, Pattison G, Stobo JB (1986) Cholera toxin inhibits the T-cell antigen receptor-mediated increases in inositol triphosphate and cytoplasmic free calcium. Proc Natl Acad Sci USA 83: 5673–5677

Johnson GL, Kaslow HR, Bourne HR (1978) Genetic evidence that cholera toxin substrates are regulatory components of adenylate cyclase. J Biol Chem 253: 7120–7123

Jones DT, Reed RR (1987) Molecular cloning of five GTP-binding protein cDNA species from rat olfactory neuroepithelium. J Biol Chem 262: 14241–14249

Jones DT, Masters SB, Bourne HR, Reed RR (1990) Biochemical characterization of three stimulatory GTP-binding proteins. J Biol Chem 265: 2671–2676

Kahn RA, Gilman AG (1984a) Purification of a protein cofactor required for ADP-ribosylation of the stimulatory regulatory component of adenylate cyclase by cholera toxin. J Biol Chem 259: 6228–6234

Kahn RA, Gilman AG (1984b) ADP-ribosylation of G_s promotes the dissociation of its α and β subunits. J Biol Chem 259: 6235–6240

Kahn RA, Gilman AG (1986) The protein cofactor necessary for ADP-ribosylation of G_s by cholera toxin is itself a GTP-binding protein. J Biol Chem 261: 7906–7911

Kahn RA, Goddard C, Newkirk M (1988) Chemical and immunological characterization of the 21-kDa ADP-ribosylation factor of adenylate cyclase. J Biol Chem 263: 8282–8287

Kelly MT (1986) Cholera: a worldwide perspective. Pediatr Infect Dis 5: S101–S105

Kimberg DV, Field M, Johnson J, Henderson A, Gershon E (1971) Stimulation of intestinal mucosal adenyl cyclase by cholera enterotoxin and prostaglandins. J Clin Invest 50: 1218–1230

Kozasa T, Itoh H, Tsukamoto T, Kaziro Y (1988) Isolation and characterization of the human $G_{s\alpha}$ gene. Proc Natl Acad Sci USA 85: 2081–2085

Kunz BC, Muczynski KA, Tsai S-C, Adamik RA, Chang PP, Moss J, Vaughan M (1990) Expression of an ADP-ribosylation factor, a GTP-dependent protein activator of cholera toxin, in the baculovirus cloning system (Abstr). FASEB J 4: A2077

Landis CA, Masters SB, Spada A, Pace AM, Bourne HR, Vallar L (1989) GTPase inhibiting mutations activate the α chain of G_s and stimulate adenylyl cyclase in human pituitary tumors. Nature 340: 692–696

Lee C-M, Chang PP, Tsai S-C, Adamik R, Price SR, Kunz BC, Moss J, Twiddy EM, Holmes RK (1991) Activation of *Escherichia coli* heat-labile enterotoxins by native and recombinant adenosine diphosphate-ribosylation factors, 20-kDa guanine nucleotide-binding proteins. J Clin Invest 87: 1780–1786

LeVine H III, Cuatrecasas P (1981) Activation of pigeon erythrocyte adenylate cyclase by cholera toxin. Partial purification of an essential macromolecular factor from horse erythrocyte cytosol. Biochim Biophys Acta 672: 248–261

Lin MC, Welton AF, Berman MF (1978) Essential role of GTP in the expression of adenylate cyclase activity after cholera toxin treatment. J Cyclic Nucleotide Res 4: 159–168

Lo WW, Hughes J (1987) A novel cholera toxin-sensitive G-protein (G_c) regulating receptor-mediated phosphoinositide signalling in human pituitary clonal cells. FEBS Lett 220: 327–331

Lochrie MA, Hurley JB, Simon MI (1985) Sequence of the alpha subunit of photoreceptor G protein: homologies between transducin, *ras*, and elongation factors. Science 228: 96–99

Maller JL, Krebs EG (1977) Progesterone-stimulated meiotic cell division in *Xenopus* oocytes. J Biol Chem 252: 1712–1718

Mattera R, Graziano MP, Yatani A, Zhou Z, Graf R, Codina J, Birnbaumer L, Gilman AG, Brown AM (1989) Splice variants of the α subunits of the G protein G_s activate both adenylyl cyclase and calcium channels. Science 243: 804–807

McCloskey MA (1988) Cholera toxin potentiates IgE-coupled inositol phospholipid hydrolysis and mediator secretion by RBL-2H3 cells. Proc Natl Acad Sci USA 85: 7260–7264

McGrath JP, Capon DJ, Goeddel DV, Levinson AD (1984) Comparative biochemical properties of normal and activated human *ras* p21 protein. Nature 310: 644–649

Medynski DC, Sullivan K, Smith D, van Dop C, Chang F-H, Fung BK-K, Seeburg PH, Bourne HR (1985) Amino acid sequence of the α subunit of transducin deduced from the cDNA sequence. Proc Natl Acad Sci USA 82: 4311–4315

Mekalanos JJ, Collier RJ, Romig WR (1979a) Enzymic activity of cholera toxin. I. New method of assay and the mechanism of ADP-ribosyl transfer. J Biol Chem 254: 5849–5854

Mekalanos JJ, Collier RJ, Romig WR (1979b) Enzymic activity of cholera toxin. II. Relationships to proteolytic processing, disulfide bond reduction, and subunit composition. J Biol Chem 254: 5855–5861

Monaco L, Murtagh JJ, Newman KB, Tsai S-C, Moss J, Vaughan M (1990) Selective amplification of an mRNA and related pseudogene for a human ADP-ribosylation factor, a guanine nucleotide-dependent protein activator of cholera toxin. Proc Natl Acad Sci USA 87: 2206–2210

Moss J, Richardson SH (1978) Activation of adenylate cyclase by heat-labile *Escherichia coli* enterotoxin. Evidence for ADP-ribosyltransferase activity similar to that of choleragen. J Clin Invest 62: 281–285

Moss J, Vaughan M (1977a) Mechanism of action of choleragen. Evidence for ADP-ribosyltransferase activity with arginine as an acceptor. J Biol Chem 252: 2455–2457

Moss J, Vaughan M (1977b) Choleragen activation of solubilized adenylate cyclase: requirement for GTP and protein activator for demonstration of enzymatic activity. Proc Natl Acad Sci USA 74: 4396–4400

Moss J, Vaughan M (1978) Isolation of an avian erythrocyte protein possessing ADP-ribosyltransferase activity and capable of activating adenylate cyclase. Proc Natl Acad Sci USA 75: 3621–3624

Moss J, Vaughan M (1988a) ADP-ribosylation of guanyl nucleotide-binding regulatory proteins by bacterial toxins. Adv Enzymol 61: 303–379

Moss J, Vaughan M (1988b) Mechanism of action of choleragen (cholera toxin) and *E. Coli* heat-labile enterotoxins. In: Tu AT, Hardegree MC (eds) Bacterial toxins. Dekker, New York (Handbook of natural toxins, vol 4)

Moss J, Vaughan M (1990) Participation of guanine nucleotide-binding protein cascade in activation of adenylyl cyclase by cholera toxin (choleragen). In: Iyengar R, Birnbaumer L (eds) G proteins. Academic, San Diego

Moss J, Manganiello VC, Vaughan M (1976) Hydrolysis of nicotinamide adenine dinucleotide by choleragen and its A protomer: possible role in the activation of adenylate cyclase. Proc Natl Acad Sci USA 73: 4424–4427

Moss J, Garrison S, Fishman PH, Richardson SH (1979a) Gangliosides sensitize unresponsive fibroblasts to *Escherichia coli* heat-labile enterotoxin. J Clin Invest 64: 381–384

Moss J, Garrison S, Oppenheimer NJ, Richardson SH (1979b) NAD-dependent ADP-ribosylation of arginine and proteins by *Escherichia coli* heat-labile enterotoxin. J Biol Chem 254: 6270–6272

Moss J, Stanley SJ, Lin MC (1979c) NAD glycohydrolase and ADP-ribosyltransferase activities are intrinsic to the A_1 peptide of choleragen. J Biol Chem 254: 11993–11996

Moss J, Stanley SJ, Watkins PA, Vaughan M (1980) ADP-ribosyltransferase activity of mono- and multi- (ADP-ribosylated) choleragen. J Biol Chem 255: 7835–7837

Moss J, Osborne JC Jr, Fishman PH, Nakaya S, Robertson DC (1981) *Escherichia coli* heat-labile enterotoxin: ganglioside specificity and ADP-ribosyltransferase activity. J Biol Chem 256: 12861–12865

Moss J, Jacobson MK, Stanley SJ (1985) Reversibility of arginine-specific mono (ADP-ribosyl)ation: identification in erythrocytes of an ADP-ribose-L-arginine cleavage enzyme. Proc Natl Acad Sci USA 82: 5603–5607

Moss J, Tsai S-C, Price SR, Bobak DA, Vaughan M (1991) Soluble guanine nucleotide-dependent ADP-ribosylation factors in activation of adenylyl cyclase by choleragen. Methods Enzymol 195: 243–256

Nakaya S, Moss J, Vaughan M (1980) Effects of nucleoside triphosphates on choleragen-activated brain adenylate cyclase. Biochemistry 19: 4871–4874

Narasimhan V, Holowka D, Fewtrell C, Baird B (1988) Cholera toxin increases the rate of antigen-stimulated calcium influx in rat basophilic leukemia cells. J Biol Chem 263: 19626–19632

Navon SE, Fung BK-K (1984) Characterization of transducin from bovine retinal rod outer segments. Mechanism and effects of cholera toxin-catalyzed ADP-ribosylation. J Biol Chem 259: 6686–6693

Noda M, Tsai S-C, Adamik R, Bobak DA, Moss J, Vaughan M (1989) Activation of immobilized, biotinylated choleragen A1 protein by a 19-kilodalton guanine nucleotide-binding protein. Biochemistry 28: 7936–7940

Noda M, Tsai S-C, Adamik R, Moss J, Vaughan M (1990) Mechanism of cholera toxin activation by a guanine nucleotide-dependent 19 kDa protein. Biochim Biophys Acta 1034: 195–199

Noda M, Tsai S-C, Adamik R, Bobak DA, Bliziotes MM, Moss J, Vaughan M (1992) Activation of cholera toxin by soluble guanine nucleotide-binding proteins. 24th US-Japan Joint Cholera Conference, Tokyo (in press)

Northup JK, Sternweis PC, Smigel MD, Schleifer LS, Ross EM, Gilman AG (1980) Purification of the regulatory component of adenylate cyclase. Proc Natl Acad Sci USA 77: 6516–6520

O'Keefe E, Cuatracasas P (1974) Cholera toxin mimics melanocyte stimulating hormone in inducing differentiation in melanoma cells. Proc Natl Acad Sci USA 71: 2500–2504

Peng Z, Calvert I, Clark J, Helman L, Kahn R, Kung H-F (1989) Molecular cloning, sequence analysis and mRNA expression of human ADP-ribosylation factor. Biofactors 2: 45–49

Peterson JW, Ochoa LG (1989) Role of prostaglandins and cAMP in the secretory effects of cholera toxin. Science 245: 857–859

Pickett CL, Holmes RK (1992) Nucleotide sequence of *Escherichia coli* heat-labile enterotoxin type IIa and IIb and comparisons to type I enterotoxin and cholera toxin. In: Advances in research in cholera and related diarrheas, vol 7. KTK, Tokyo (in press)

Pickett CL, Twiddy EM, Belisle BW, Holmes RK (1986) Cloning of genes that encode a new heat-labile enterotoxin of *Escherichia coli*. J Bacteriol 165: 348–352

Pickett CL, Weinstein DL, Holmes RK (1987) Genetics of type IIa heat-labile enterotoxin of *Escherichia coli*: operon fusions, nucleotide sequence, and hybridization studies. J Bacteriol 169: 5180–5187

Pickett CL, Twiddy EM, Coker C, Holmes RK (1989) Cloning, nucleotide sequence, and hybridization studies of the type IIb heat-labile enterotoxin gene of *Escherichia coli*. J Bacteriol 171: 4945–4952

Pierce NF (1973) Differential inhibitory effects of cholera toxoids and ganglioside on the enterotoxins of *Vibrio cholerae* and *Escherichia coli*. J Exp Med 137: 1009–1023

Pike LJ, Eakes AT (1987) Epidermal growth factor stimulates the production of phosphatidylinositol monophosphate and the breakdown of polyphosphoinositides in A431 cells. J Biol Chem 262: 1644–1651

Pinkett MO, Anderson WB (1982) Plasma membrane-associated component(s) that confer(s) cholera toxin sensitivity to adenylate cyclase. Biochim Biophys Acta 714: 337–343

Price SR, Nightingale M, Tsai S-C, Williamson KC, Adamik R, Chen H-C, Moss J, Vaughan M (1988) Guanine nucleotide-binding proteins that enhance choleragen ADP-ribosyltransferase activity: nucleotide and deduced amino acid sequence of an ADP-ribosylation factor cDNA. Proc Natl Acad Sci USA 85: 5488–5491

Price SR, Barber A, Moss J (1990) Structure-function relationships of guanine nucleotide-binding proteins. In: Moss J, Vaughan M (eds) ADP-ribosylating toxins and G proteins: insights into signal transduction. American Society for Microbiology, Washington

Robertson DC, Kunkel SL, Galligan PH (1980) Structure and function of *E. coli* heat-labile enterotoxin. 15th Joint Conference on Cholera, (DHEW publ no (NIH) 80–2003)

Robishaw JD, Russell DW, Harris BA, Smigel MD, Gilman AG (1986a) Deduced primary structure of the α subunit of the GTP-binding stimulatory protein of adenylate cyclase. Proc Natl Acad Sci USA 83: 1251–1255

Robishaw JD, Smigel MD, Gilman AG (1986b) Molecular basis for two forms of the G protein that stimulates adenylate cyclase. J Biol Chem 261: 9587–9590

Rothman JE, Orci L (1990) Movement of proteins through the Golgi stack: a molecular dissection of vesicular transport. FASEB J 4: 1460–1468

Salminen A, Novick PJ (1987) A *ras*-like protein is required for a post-Golgi event in yeast secretion. Cell 49: 527–538

Sattler J, Schwarzmann G, Knack I, Röhm R-H, Wiegandt H (1978) Studies of ligand binding to cholera toxin. III. Cooperativity of oligosaccharide binding. Hoppe Seylers Z Physiol Chem 359: 719–723

Schleifer LS, Kahn RA, Hanski E, Northup JK, Sternweis PC, Gilman AG (1982) Requirements for cholera toxin-dependent ADP-ribosylation of the purified regulatory component of adenylate cyclase. J Biol Chem 257: 20–23

Schmidt GJ, Huber LJ, Weiter JJ (1987) A-protein catalyzes the ADP-ribosylation of G-protein from cow rod outer segments. J Biol Chem 262: 14333–14336

Schwarzmann G, Mraz W, Sattler J, Schinder R, Wiegandt H (1978) Comparison of the interaction of mono- and oligovalent ligands with cholera toxin—demonstration of aggregate formation at low ligand concentrations. Hoppe Seylers Z Physiol Chem 359: 1277–1286

Segev N, Mulholland J, Botstein D (1988) The yeast GTP-binding YPT1 protein and a mammalian counterpart are associated with the secretion machinery. Cell 52: 915–924

Sewell JL, Kahn RA (1988) Sequences of the bovine and yeast ADP-ribosylation factor and comparison to other GTP-binding proteins. Proc Natl Acad Sci USA 85: 4620–4624

Stearns T, Willingham MC, Botstein D, Kahn RA (1990a) ADP-ribosylation factor is functionally and physically associated with the Golgi complex. Proc Natl Acad Sci USA 87: 1238–1242

Stearns T, Kahn RA, Botstein D, Hoyt MA (1990b) ADP ribosylation factor is an essential protein in *Saccharomyces cerevisiae* and is encoded by two genes. Mol Cell Biol 10: 6690–6699

Stryer L, Bourne HR (1986) G proteins: a family of signal transducers. Annu Rev Cell Biol 2: 391–419

Sweet RW, Yokoyama S, Kamata T, Feramisco JR, Rosenberg M, Gross M (1984) The product of *ras* is a GTPase and the T24 oncogenic mutant is deficient in this activity. Nature 311: 273–275

Tanabe T, Nukada T, Nishikawa Y, Sugimoto K, Suzuki H, Takahashi H, Noda M, Haga T, Ichiyama A, Kangawa K, Minamino N, Matsuo H, Numa S (1985) Primary structure of the α-subunit of transducin and its relationship to *ras* proteins. Nature 315: 242–245

Towler DA, Eubanks SR, Towery DS, Adams SP, Glaser L (1987) Amino-terminal processing of proteins by N-myristoylation. J Biol Chem 262: 1030–1036

Trahey M, McCormick F (1987) A cytoplasmic protein stimulates normal N-*ras* p21 GTPase, but does not affect oncogenic mutants. Science 238: 542–545

Trepel JB, Chuang D-M, Neff NH (1977) Transfer of ADP-ribose from NAD to choleragen: a subunit acts as catalyst and acceptor protein. Proc Natl Acad Sci USA 74: 5440–5442

Tsai S-C, Noda M, Adamik R, Moss J, Vaughan M (1987) Enhancement of choleragen ADP-ribosyltransferase activities by guanyl nucleotides and a 19-kDa membrane protein. Proc Natl Acad Sci USA 84: 5139–5142

Tsai S-C, Noda M, Adamik R, Chang PP, Chen H-C, Moss J, Vaughan M (1988) Stimulation of choleragen enzymatic activities by GTP and two soluble proteins purified from bovine brain. J Biol Chem 263: 1768–1772

Tsai S-C, Adamik R, Moss J, Vaughan M (1991a) Guanine nucleotide-dependent formation of a complex between choleragen (cholera toxin) A subunit and bovine brain ADP-ribosylation factor. Biochemistry 30: 3697–3703

Tsai S-C, Adamik R, Tsuchiya M, Chang PP, Moss J, Vaughan M (1991b) Differential expression during development of ADP-ribosylation factors, 20-kDa guanine nucleotide-binding protein activators of cholera toxin. J Biol Chem 266: 8213–8219

Tsuchiya M, Price SR, Nightingale MS, Moss J, Vaughan M (1989) Tissue and species distribution of mRNA encoding two ADP-ribosylation factors, 20-kDa guanine nucleotide binding proteins. Biochemistry 28: 9668–9673

Tsuchiya M, Price SR, Tsai S-C, Moss J, Vaughan M (1991) Molecular identification of ADP-ribosylation factor mRNAs and their expression in mammalian cells. J Biol Chem 266: 2772–2777

Van Dop C, Tsubokawa M, Bourne HR, Ramachandran J (1984) Amino acid sequence of retinal transducin at the site ADP-ribosylated by cholera toxin. J Biol Chem 259: 696–698

Van Heyningen WE, Carpenter CCJ, Pierce NF, Greenough WB III (1971) Deactivation of cholera toxin by ganglioside. J Infect Dis 124: 415–418

Vaughan M, Tsai S-C, Noda M, Adamik R, Moss J (1989) Participation of a guanine nucleotide-binding protein cascade in cholera toxin activation of adenylate cyclase. J Mol Cell Cardiol [Suppl 1] 21: 97–102

Watkins PA, Moss J, Vaughan M (1980) Effects of GTP on choleragen-catalyzed ADP ribosylation of membrane and soluble proteins. J Biol Chem 255: 3959–3963

Weiss O, Holden J, Rulka C, Kahn RA (1989) Nucleotide binding and cofactor activities of purified bovine brain and bacterially expressed ADP-ribosylation factor. J Biol Chem 264: 21066–21072

Woolkalis M, Gill DM, Coburn J (1988) Assay and purification of cytosolic factor required for cholera toxin activity. Methods Enzymol 165: 246–249

Yatani A, Imoto Y, Codina J, Hamilton S, Brown AM, Birnbaumer L (1988) The stimulatory G protein of adenylyl cyclase, G_s, also stimulates dihydropyridine-sensitive Ca^{++} channels. J Biol Chem 263: 9887–9895

Yatsunami K, Khorana HG (1985) GTPase of bovine rod outer segments: the amino acid sequence of the α subunit as derived from the cDNA sequence. Proc Natl Acad Sci USA 82: 4316–4320

ADP-Ribosylation of Signal-Transducing Guanine Nucleotide-Binding Proteins by Pertussis Toxin

P. GIERSCHIK

1 Introduction

The gram-negative bacterium *Bordetella pertussis*, the causative agent of whooping cough, produces a number of virulence factors, among which pertussis toxin is undoubtedly of major importance (WEISS and HEWLETT 1986). Pertussis toxin elicits a myriad of biological effects in patients suffering from whooping cough or infected laboratory animals and has thus received several names, including histamine-sensitizing factor, lymphocytosis-promoting factor, islet-activating protein (IAP), or simply pertussigen.

Whooping cough is a major health problem affecting some 60 million patients and causing about 1 million deaths per year. The disease can, in principle, be prevented by vaccination. However, the use of the classical vaccine (chemically inactivated *B. pertussis* cells) is associated with convulsions (1: 1750), and even severe and permanent neurologic damage (1: 310000) (CODY et al. 1981; MILLER et al. 1984). Among the various components in the classical vaccine is pertussis toxin, which appears to contain an important

Pharmakologisches Institut, Universität Heidelberg, Im Neuenheimer Feld 366, 6900 Heidelberg, FRG

Current Topics in Microbiology and Immunology, Vol. 175

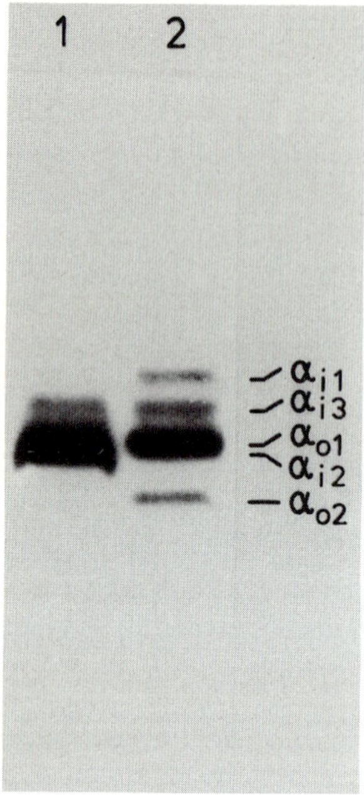

Fig. 1. ADP-ribosylation of human G protein α-subunits by pertussis toxin. Membrane proteins of myeloid differentiated human leukemia (HL-60) cells (*lane 1*) and human brain (*lane 2*) were treated with dithiothreitol-activated pertussis toxin and [^{32}P]NAD$^+$. Subsequently, the samples were subjected to SDS/Urea-PAGE see GIERSCHIK et al. 1989a, for experimental details) and autoradiography was performed. The positions of the [^{32}P]ADP-ribosylated α-subunits are indicated on the right. HL-60 membranes contain two pertussis toxin substrate (α_{i2} and α_{i3}). At least four substrates are present in human brain membranes (see Table 1 for further information)

epitope that leads to the formation of antibodies capable of protecting against disease (SATO et al. 1984; 1987; BARTOLONI et al. 1988; KIM et al. 1989; DE MAGISTRIS et al. 1989; ASKELÖF et al. 1990). The latter ovservation prompted large-scale clinical trials using chemically detoxified pertussis toxin as immunogen (AD HOC GROUP FOR THE STUDY OF PERTUSSIS VACCINES 1988). Although this regimen turned out to be quite efficacious in preventing whooping cough, the acellular vaccines remained associated with uncertainties about their safety (AD HOC GROUP FOR THE STUDY OF PERTUSSIS VACCINES 1988; STORSAETER et al. 1988). To solve this problem, several research groups have turned their attention towards examining the molecular properties of pertussis toxin. This work not only resulted in the development of very promising candidates for a safer, genetically detoxified vaccine against whooping cough (PIZZA et al. 1989), but also led to an enormous increase in the knowledge of the architecture and molecular mechanisms of action of pertussis toxin.

The great majority of the biological effects of pertussis toxin are due to a toxin-catalyzed transfer of an adenosine diphosphate an (ADP)-ribose moiety from NAD$^+$ to the α-subunits of a certain subset of the family of signal-transducing guanine-nucleotide-binding proteins (G proteins). ADP-ribosylation generally leads to an uncoupling of the modified G protein from the corresponding receptor. It is this property that has made pertussis toxin an extremely important tool for investigators involved in signal transduction research, since the toxin can be used (a) to selectively alter the function of specific G proteins by treating intact cells or membrane preparations with the toxin and NAD^+, and (b) to selectively radiolavel and thus identify G protein α-subunits in crude membrane preparations using [^{32}P]ADP-ribosylation followed by analysis of the modified proteins by sodium dodecyl sulfate-polyacrylamide gel electrophoresis (see Fig. 1 for an example of such an analysis).

Four aspects of the structure and function of pertussis toxin are reviewed here: (a) the structure of the toxin and the structure–function relationships of its enzymatically active S1 subunit, (b) the main structural and functional properties of pertussis-toxin-sensitive G proteins, (c) the molecular mechanisms of pertussis toxin-mediated G protein ADP-ribosylation, and (d) the functional consequences elicited by this modification. Given the limited space, I have not been able to provide a complete overview of the literature on these topics. The reader is referred to several excellent previous reviews and monographs on pertussis toxin for more complete information (UI 1984, 1986; SEKURA et al. 1985; MOSS and VAUGHAN 1988; MANCLARK 1990).

2 Structure of Pertussis Toxin

Pertussis toxin is a 105-kDa hexameric protein composed of five distinct noncovalently linked polypeptides designated (in the order of decreasing molecular weight) S1–S5 (Fig. 2). Pertussis toxin can be divided into two distinct functional units, the enzymatically active A-protomer consisting of a single polypeptide (S1), and the pentameric B-oligomer (S2, S3, two copies of S4, and S5). The B-oligomer is involved in binding to the surface of eukaryotic target cells and presumably in translocation of the toxin across the plasma membrane (TAMURA et al. 1982, 1983; BRENNAN et al. 1988; WITVLIET et al. 1989). The two S4 polypeptides form two distinct heterodimers with S2 and S3 (S2–S4 and S3–S4), which are in turn held together by S5 (TAMURA et al. 1982) The site(s) of interaction of S1 with the B-oligomer is unknown.

The genes coding for the pertussis toxin subunits have been cloned and sequenced (NICOSIA et al. 1986; LOCHT et al. 1986; LOCHT and KEITH 1986). The five genes are arranged in tandem and form a single operon. All subunits contain signal peptides of variable length. The calculated molecular weights of the mature subunits are 26 220 (235 amino acids) for S1, 21 920 (199 amino acids) for S2, 21 860 (199 amino acids) for S3, 12 060 (110 amino acids) for S4, and 10 940 (99 amino acids) for S5 (NICOSIA et al. 1986). Two distinct sequences have been published for S1, differing in the region from amino acids 190–200. As the S1 sequence published by NICOSIA et al. (1986) has been independently confirmed by others (M.A. Schmidt, ZMBH, Heidelberg, personal communication; PIZZA et al. 1991), I will use this sequence for further reference.

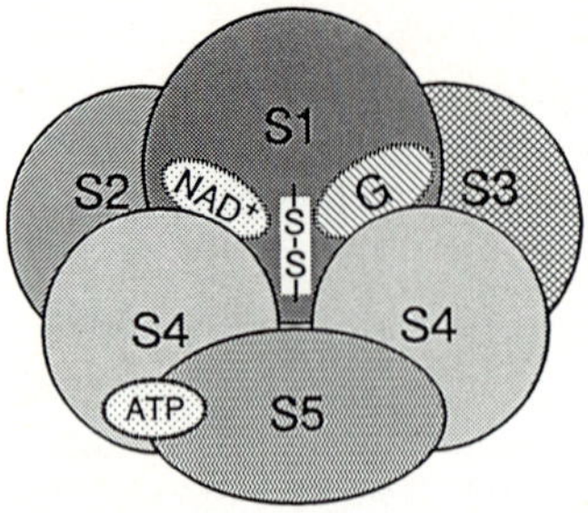

Fig. 2. Subunit structure of pertussis toxin. Pertussis toxin is composed of six subunits. S1 is the enzymatically active subunit and contains the binding site for NAD^+ and the G protein substrates (G). The remainder of the molecule (the two dimers S4–S3 and S4–S2, and the connecting subunit S5) is responsible for binding of the toxin to the target cell (B-oligomer). Reduction of the intra-molecular disulfide bond of S1 and binding of ATP to the B-oligomer leads to release of S1 from the B-oligomer and S1 activation. See text for further details

3 Structure–Function Relationships of the S1 Subunit of Pertussis Toxin

The S1 subunit of pertussis toxin harbors two enzymatic activities: (a) an ADP-ribosyltransferase activity that catalyzes the transfer of an ADP-ribose moiety from NAD^+ to a cysteine localized three amino acids upstream of the carboxy-terminal residue of the α-subunits of various heterotrimeric G proteins (see below) or even to free cysteine (LOBBAN and VAN HEYNINGEN 1988), and (b) a NAD^+ glycohydrolase activity that hydrolyzes NAD^+ to ADP-ribose and nicotinamide and is operative in the absence of a suitable acceptor (KATADA et al. 1983; MOSS et al. 1983). The enzymatic activity of S1 is silent in both the native A-protomer (KATADA et al. 1983) and in the holotoxin (MOSS et al. 1983), and is synergistically activated in vitro by a variety of substances, including sulfhydryl agents, adenine nucleotides, certain phospholipids and detergents (KATADA et al. 1983; MOSS et al. 1983, 1986; KASLOW et al. 1987). Cellular glutathione (possibly in conjunction with a thiol: protein disulfide oxidoreductase; MOSS et al. 1980, adenosine triphosphate (ATP), and membrane lipids of the toxin target cells may be the relevant activators in vivo (KASLOW et al. 1987).

S1 contains two cysteine residues, in positions 41 and 201, which are disulfide bonded in the native toxin (SEKURA et al. 1983). Reduction of this disulfide bond by dithiothreitol leads to a marked stimulation of S1 activity, which coincides with a release of S1 from the B-oligomer (BURNS and MANCLARK 1989). Alkylation or deletion by site-directed mutagenesis of Cys^{41} (but not of Cys^{201}) markedly reduces the NAD^+ glycohydrolase and the ADP-ribosyltransferase activity of S1 (KASLOW and LESIKAR 1987; KASLOW et al. 1989; BURNS and MANCLARK 1989; LOCHT et al. 1990). It is of interest to note that recombinant, truncated S1 polypeptides lacking Cys^{201} still require millimolar concentrations of dithiothreitol in order to express maximal NAD^+ glycohydrolase and ADP-ribosyltransferase activity (LOCHT et al. 1990; LOCHT and CABEZON 1990;

CORTINA et al. 1991). As the truncated proteins do not appear to dimerize in the absence of dithiothreitol (LOCHT et al. 1990; LOCHT and CABEZON 1990; CORTINA et al. 1991), it has been suggested that Cys^{41} may be modified by an unknown small molecular weight moiety in this case (LOCHT and CABEZON 1990). Replacement of Cys^{41} by a variety of amino acids reveals that the side chain of Cys^{41} is not absolutely necessary for the catalytic functions of S1 (KASLOW et al. 1989; LOCHT et al. 1990). Thus, Cys^{41} is very likely to be located close to the NAD^+ binding site of S1 and may be an important determinant of the affinity of the S1–NAD^+ interaction. The detrimental effect of replacing Cys^{41} with negatively charged residues suggests that Cys^{41} is located close to at least one of the phosphates of NAD^+ (LOCHT et al. 1990).

Adenine nucleotides facilitate activation of pertussis toxin by interacting with the B-oligomer (MOSS et al. 1986; BURNS and MANCLARK 1986; HAUSMAN et al. 1990). This activation is probably due to the ATP-induced release of S1 from the B-oligomer (BURNS and MANCLARK 1986). It is of interest that ATP actually inhibits both the NAD^+ glycohydrolase and the ADP-ribosyltransferase activity of the recombinant (i.e., free) S1 polypeptide (CORTINA and BARBIERI 1991). Although ATP is clearly the most effective and potent nucleotide activator of the holotoxin, activation can also be elicited with ADP, other nucleoside di- and triphosphates, or even inorganic polyphosphates (MOSS et al. 1986; KASLOW et al. 1987; MATTERA et al. 1986, 1987). Note that inorganic monophosphates do not elicit toxin activation, but even inhibit G-protein ADP-ribosylation by the toxin (KASLOW et al. 1987; RIBEIRO-NETO et al. 1987). The latter effect is almost certainly due to an inhibition by monophosphates of the binding of adenine or guanine nucleotides to the toxin (MATTERA et al. 1986; HAUSMAN et al. 1990). Taken together, these results strongly suggest that ATP promotes pertussis toxin activation via its phosphate groups and that the adenine moiety is important for the high-affinity interaction of the nucleotide with the B-oligomer.

The ability of ATP to facilitate dithiothreitol-mediated toxin activation is markedly enhanced in the presence of phospholipids and certain ionic and nonionic detergents (MOSS et al. 1986; KASLOW et al. 1987). Interestingly, the ability of certain detergents, e.g., 3-[(3-cholamidopropyl) dimethylammanio]-1-propane sulfonate (CHAPS), to stimulate NAD^+ glycohydrolysis does not correlate with their effect on ADP-ribosyltransferase activity (MOSS et al. 1986). Presumably, these detergents have additional effects on the ADP-ribose acceptor (see also RIBEIRO-NETO et al. 1987; HODGES et al. 1989). The site of interaction of lipophilic substances with the toxin has been mapped to S1 (MOSS et al. 1986). Surprisingly, this site does not appear to be located within the hydrophobic C-terminus (residues 188–235, see below), as CHAPS markedly stimulates NAD^+ hydrolysis by a truncated hydrophilic S1 subunit expressed in *Escherichia coli* (LOCHT et al. 1989). Thus, lipophilic substances may affect toxin activation through mechanisms other than increasing solubility.

In addition to Cys^{41}, at least four other residues have been identified to be critical for S1 function, i.e., Arg^9, Arg^{13}, Trp^{26}, and Glu^{129}. Substitution of Arg^9

with Lys, or Arg^{13} with either Leu or Lys leads to a marked reduction of ADP-ribosyltransferase activity (BURNETTE et al. 1988; PIZZA et al. 1989). An S1 protein carrying mutations in both positions displays ADP-ribosyltransferase activity which is at least 10000-fold lower than that of the native S1 protein (PIZZA et al. 1989). Interestingly, both Arg^{9} and Arg^{13} lie within a stretch of eight amino acids which are nearly identical in sequence to similarly located regions of cholera and *E. coli* heat-labile toxin (see below). This suggests that all three toxins may interact with NAD^{+} via this very homologous region (LOCHT and KEITH 1986).

A Glu-X-X-X-X-Trp motif has been known for quite some time to be important for the interaction of both diphtheria toxin and *Pseudomonas aeruginosa* exotoxin A (toxins which ADP-ribosylate elongation factor 2) with the nicotinamide moiety of NAD^{+} (for further information see CARROLL and COLLIER 1987; WILSON and COLLIER, this volume). Recent evidence suggests that Glu^{129} and Trp^{26} fulfill similar functions in the S1 subunit of pertussis toxin and that the protein folding provides for the appropriate spacing of the two residues in the native S1 protein (PIZZA et al. 1988; BARBIERI and CORTINA 1988; LOCHT et al. 1989; CORTINA and BARBIERI 1989). Of interest in this regard is that Glu^{129} has recently been shown to serve substrate for photolabeling with NAD^{+} (BARBIERI et al. 1989; COCKLE 1989; CIEPLAK et al. 1990). By analogy to similar studies performed with diphtheria toxin and *Pseudomonas aeruginosa* exotoxin A, these results suggest that the number 6 carbon atom of the NAD^{+} nicotinamide moiety comes into close proximity of the γ-methylene group of Glu^{129} (CARROLL et al. 1985; CARROLL and COLLIER 1987). Thus, Glu^{129} is located within or at least very close to the catalytic centre of the S1 subunit.

The knowledge of structurally important residues of S1 summarized above together with immunological data and results from structure–function studies

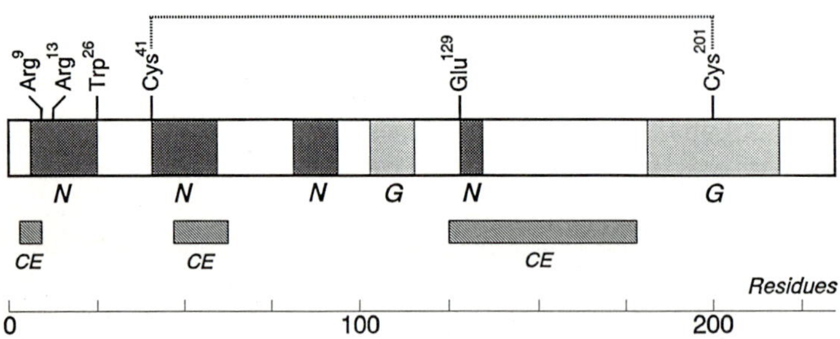

Fig. 3. Model for the organization of the S1 subunit of pertussis toxin into functional domains. The sites of interaction of S1 with NAD^{+} (*N*), the G protein (*G*), and the conformational epitope (*CE*) reactive with a panel of monoclonal antibodies used by BARTOLONI et al. (1988) are shown. The sites for interaction with NAD^{+} are inferred from (a) the knowledge of functionally important residues (see text), (b) comparison of the amino acid sequences of S1 and the A1 subunit of cholera toxin (DOMENIGHINI et al. 1991), and (c) comparison of the primary structure of the NAD^{+} binding site of *E. coli* heat-labile enterotoxin (SIXMA et al. 1991) and the amino acid sequence of S1

utilizing truncated S1 mutants allow us to construct a tentative structural model for the S1 protein. A schematic representation of this model is shown in Fig. 3. Deletion mapping showed that residues 2 through 179 possess both NAD^+ glycohydrolase and ADP-ribosyltransferase activities (LOCHT et al. 1987; PIZZA et al. 1988; BARBIERI et al. 1989b), although the latter activity appears to be present at a much lower level in C-terminally truncated S1 proteins than in the wild type protein (LOCHT et al. 1990; CORTINA and BARBIERI 1991; see below). Arg^9, Arg^{13}, Trp^{26}, Cys^{41}, and Glu^{129} are likely to be located close to the NAD^+ substrate, indicating that these residues come close to each other in the native, activated S1 protein. This view is supported by the finding that three regions (i.e., those encompassing residues 2–10, $\approx 45-\approx 65$, and 124–179) are required to form the immunodominant conformational epitope recognized by seven protective monoclonal antibodies raised against S1 (BARTOLONI et al. 1988). Furthermore, replacement of Glu^{129} by a cysteine residue led to formation of a disulfide bind between Cys^{129} and Cys^{41}, suggesting that Glu^{129} and Cys^{41} lie in close proximity in the activated S1 polypeptide (LOCHT and CABEZON 1990). The hydrophobic C-terminus is important for the binding of S1 to the B-oligomer. This interaction is likely to be crucial for the assembly of the holotoxin and its secretion from the periplasmic space of the bacterium (BURNS et al. 1987; BURNS and MANCLARK 1989; ANTOINE and LOCHT 1990; PIZZA et al. 1990).

The S1 polypeptide appears to contain at least two domains necessary for interaction with the G protein. One of these has recently been mapped to an area between residues 181 and 219 (CORTINA and BARBIERI 1991). A second domain has been postulated to be located between residues 2 and 179, since truncated S1 proteins encompassing these residues are clearly capable of ADP-ribosylating the G protein substrate, albeit less efficiently than wild type S1 (LOCHT et al. 1987; PIZZA et al. 1988; BARBIERI et al. 1989b; LOCHT et al. 1990; CORTINA and BARBIERI 1991). The precise location of this second domain is unknown. A potential candidate, however, is the area around residue 110. This suggestion is based on (a) the observation that replacement of Tyr^{111} with Gly together with an insertion of a tetrapeptide in position 113 *enhances*, while insertion of four additional amino acids in position 107 markedly *reduces* ADP-ribosyltransferase activity of S1 (PIZZA et al. 1988; BLACK et al. 1988), and (b) on the assumption that this area is not involved in NAD^+ binding and hydrolysis. As will be discussed below, both α- and $\beta\gamma$-subunits of the G protein are required for ADP-ribosylation of the α-subunit by activated S1. It is not known whether S1 physically interacts with both subunits. It is tempting to speculate, however, that the two-site interaction of S1 with the G protein substrate may reflect an interaction of an N-terminal S1-domain with the G protein α-subunit and the hydrophobic C-terminal domain of S1 with the hydrophobic G protein $\beta\gamma$-dimer.

4 Similarities Between the S1 Subunit of Pertussis Toxin and the A1 Chains of Cholera Toxin and *E. coli* Heat-Labile Enterotoxin

In 1986, protein chemical analysis and complementary deoxyribonucleic acid (cDNA) sequencing revealed that the N-terminal region of S1 subunit of pertussis toxin is very homologous to the N-termini of cholera toxin and *E. coli* heat-labile enterotoxin (CAPIAU et al. 1986; LOCHT and KEITH 1986; NICOSIA et al. 1986). The latter two proteins, which are known to be capable of ADP-ribosylating the α-subunits of the stimulatory G protein of adenylyl cyclase G_s, but also other α-subunits (see below) are remarkably similar in their primary structure (87% identical amino acid residues) (YAMAMOTO et al. 1984). No significant sequence homology was detected between S1 and diphtheria toxin or *Pseudomonas aeruginosa* exotoxin A. A recent, more detailed sequence comparison between S1 and the two A1 chains showed that the degree of homology between the three ADP-ribosyltransferases is actually higher than initially reported (DOMENIGHINI et al. 1991). In this report, the regions of S1 encompassing residues 1–22, 23–38, 47–65, 83–97, and 113–143 were found to be homologous to similarly located regions of the two A1 subunits. As noted earlier, Arg^{9} and Arg^{13} are perfectly aligned with Arg^{10} and Arg^{14} of the two A1 polypeptides. In contrast, no corresponding residues could be found for Trp^{26}, Cys^{41}, or Glu^{129}, suggesting that either different residues of the A1 subunits exert the functions of these important S! residues, or that Trp, Cys, and Glu residues are present at different positions of the A1 proteins to fulfill these functions.

Very recently, the crystal structure of the porcine *E. coli* heat-labile enterotoxin was reported (SIXMA et al. 1991). The structure revealed that Glu^{112} of the A1 subunits corresponds to Glu^{129} of S1. Interestingly, the three-dimensional structure of the active site of the crystalized A1 subunit is very similar to those of diphtheria toxin or *Pseudomonas aeruginosa* exotoxin A, despite the fact that there is minimal sequence homology (3 out of 44 residues).

It is clear from these studies that amino acid sequence comparisons between the different ADP-ribosyltransferases are of limited value in trying to understand the structural relationships between these proteins. Clearly, the crystal structure of S1 is required to fully understand the structure–function relationships of S1, and the degree of structural homology between the various ADP-ribosylating enzymes. These are already indications in the literature that this approach is feasible (RAGHVAAN et al. 1991).

5 Important Structural and Functional Properties of Pertussis-Toxin-Sensitive G Proteins

G proteins are key elements of many transmembrane signaling systems. G proteins function at the level of the plasma membrane and couple a great number (possibly more than 1000, see BARINAGA 1991) of receptors for extracellular mediators such as hormones, neurotransmitters, growth factors, chemoattractants, pheromones, and odorants or even physical signals such as light to effector moieties, which generate a "second message" inside the cell. The list of G-protein-regulated effectors includes enzymes, e.g., adenylyl cyclase, various phospholipases, and phosphodiesterase(s), ion channels e.g., K^+ and Ca^{2+} channels, and possibly various types of pumps, transporters, and antiporters as well (for recent reviews and references see BIRNBAUMER 1990; BIRNBAUMER et al. 1990; GIERSCHIK et al. 1990a).

G proteins are heterotrimeric proteins consisting of an α-subunit ($\approx$ 39–52 kDa) that reversibly associates with a tight complex composed of a β- and a γ-subunit ($\approx$ 36 and $\approx$ 9 kDa, respectively). The α-subunit carries the binding site for guanine nucleotides and is capable of hydrolyzing guanosine triphosphate (GTP). Biochemical and molecular biological studies have revealed all three G protein subunits are members of large protein families. Thus, messenger ribonucleic acids (mRNAs) for at least 20 different α-subunits have been identified in mammalian cells to date (LOCHRIE and SIMON 1988; HSU et al. 1990; STRATHMANN et al. 1989; STRATHMANN and SIMON 1990; JIANG et al. 1991; SIMON et al. 1991). Furthermore, there is a minimum of four distinct β-subunits (SIMON et al. 1991), and four, possibly even seven, γ-subunits (GAUTAM et al. 1990; TAMIR et al. 1991). In some cases, the molecular diversity of the α-subunits is due to alternative splicing of a single precursor RNA. For example, there are four variants of α_s and two variants of α_o (an α-subunit abundant in the brain), which are derived from a single α_s or α_o gene, respectively (BRAY et al. 1986; HSU et al. 1990; STRATHMANN et al. 1990; BERTRAND et al. 1990; TSUKAMOTO et al. 1991). On the other hand, three genes exists in the mammalian genome which encode α_i proteins. G_i proteins were initially believed to be specifically involved in inhibition of adenylyl cyclase (and hence termed G_i), but are now known to be involved in regulating other effectors as well (see BIRNBAUMER 1991; BIRNBAUMER et al. 1990; GIERSCHIK et al. 1990b, for recent reviews and references).

Many G protein α-subunits are myristoylated at an N-terminal glycine residue (BUSS et al. 1987; SCHULTZ et al. 1987; KAHN et al. 1988; MUMBY et al. 1990a; see GORDON et al. 1991, for a recent review on protein N-myristoylation). All three α_i proteins and α_o (very likely both subtypes) are myristoylated in vivo. The purified α-subunit of retinal rod transducin (α_{tr}) and the α-subunits of G_s do not appear to be myristoylated (BUSS et al. 1987). Attachment of myristate to the N-terminus of α_{o1} and α_{i1} is important for the interaction of these α-subunits with the plasma membrane (MUMBY et al. 1990a; JONES et al. 1990). Recent evidence suggests that myristoylation of α_{o1} also increases its affinity

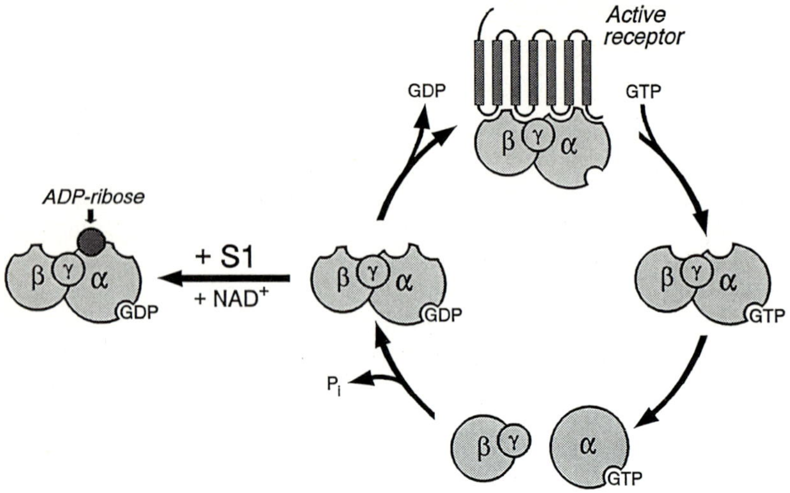

Fig. 4. Model for the activation of G proteins by receptors and its inhibition by pertussis toxin-mediated G protein ADP-ribosylation. The active receptor catalyzes the exchange of GTP for GDP bound to the quiescent heterotrimeric G protein. Binding of GTP triggers the release of the G protein from the receptor as well as its own dissociation into $\beta\gamma$-dimer and GTP-liganded α-subunit. Deactivation is initiated by hydrolysis by the α-subunit of bound GTP to GDP, which leads to reassociation of the $\alpha \cdot \beta\gamma$ heterotrimer. The G protein is most readily ADP-ribosylated by the activated S1 subunit in its GDP-bound, heterotrimeric state. Note that the site for ADP-ribosylation is not available when the unliganded G protein is bound to the active receptor. See text for further details

for $\beta\gamma$-subunits (LINDER et al. 1990). This observation led to the suggestion that myristoylation may target α_i and α_o proteins to the plasma membrane by facilitating the formation of the heterotrimer.

G protein γ-subunits also undergo post-translational modification. In this case, the processing occurs at the C-terminus and involves proteolytic removal of the last three amino acids, carboxymethylation and isoprenylation of the C-terminal cysteine (FUNG et al. 1990; BACKLUND et al. 1990; FUKADA et al. 1990; MUMBY et al. 1990b; YAMANE et al. 1990; LAI et al. 1990; MALTESE and ROBISHAW 1990; see MALTESE 1990, for a recent review of protein isoprenylation). The γ-subunit of retinal transducin has been shown to be farnesylated (FUKADA et al. 1990; LAI et al. 1990). In contrast, nonretinal γ-subunits are modified by attachment of a geranylgeranyl moiety (MUMBY et al. 1990b; YAMANE et al. 1990). The carboxy terminal processing on nonretinal γ-subunits is important for the targeting of $\beta\gamma$-subunits to the plasma membrane (SIMONDS et al. 1991). Modification of the retinal γ-subunit has been suggested to be required for $\alpha \cdot \beta\gamma$-interaction (FUKADA et al. 1989, 1990; OHGURO et al. 1990; see below).

The G-protein-mediated activation or inhibition of an effector moiety by an agonist-activated receptor is thought to result from a series of sequential interactions of receptor, G protein, and effector (Fig. 4). First, the activated receptor interacts with the heterotrimeric G protein and facilitates an exchange of GTP for guanosine diphosphate (GDP) bound to its α-subunit (FERGUSON et al. 1986). Activation of the GTP-bound form of the G protein appears to coincide with its dissociation from the receptor as well as its own dissociation into a free α-subunit and the $\beta\gamma$-dimer (IYENGAR et al. 1988; RANSNÄS and INSEL 1988). In certain cases (e.g. stimulation of adenylyl cyclase) the free GTP-bound α-subunit is responsible for effector regulation (NORTHUP et al. 1983b). In other cases, however, free $\beta\gamma$-dimers may also be directly involved in controlling effector activity (see NEER and CLAPHAM 1990, for further information). Deactivation of the G protein is thought to mainly result from the hydrolysis of bound GTP to GDP, and the subsequent association of the GDP-bound α-subunit with the $\beta\gamma$-dimer.

A very important property of G proteins in their ability to undergo ADP-ribosylation by pertussis and cholera toxin, and by the less commonly used heat-labile enterotoxin of *E. coli*. The natural and most readily modified substrates of cholera toxin (and of *E. coli* heat-labile enterotoxin) are the α-subunits of G_s. In addition, an α_s-related protein found in olfactory epithelium (termed α_{olf}) is also modified by cholera toxin (JONES and REED 1989; JONES et al. 1990). Maximal ADP-ribosylation of α_s and α_{olf} requires the presence of an additional GTP-binding protein termed ADP-ribosylation factor (ARF) (see Moss et al., this volume). ADP-ribosylation of α_s by cholera toxin inhibits its GTPase activity and thereby leads to a long-lived activation of the protein (CASSEL and SELINGER 1977; CASSEL et al. 1977). The α-subunits of several other G proteins, including retinal rod transducin and members of the G_i/G_o subfamily, are also ADP-ribosylated by cholera toxin, in particular in the presence of an activated receptor and the poorly hydrolyzable GTP analog guanosine-5′-(β,γ-imino)triphosphate (GppNHp) (ABOOD et al. 1982; NAVON and FUNG 1984; GIERSCHIK and JAKOBS 1987; GIERSCHIK et al. 1988a; IIRI et al. 1989; MILLIGAN and MCKENZIE 1988; KLINZ and COSTA 1989; MILLIGAN 1989; MILLIGAN et al. 1991). Whether or not an ARF-like protein is involved in supporting the ADP-ribosylation of the latter G proteins is unknown.

The peptide ADP-ribosylated by cholera toxin in α_{tr} has been identified by direct sequencing as Ser-Arg-Val-Lys, with Arg being the modified amino acid residue (VAN DOP et al. 1984a). Comparison of this peptide sequence with the complete amino acid sequence of α_{tr} predicted by the α_{tr} cDNA sequence (see LOCHRIE and SIMON 1988, for references) revealed that cholera toxin ADP-ribosylates an arginine residue in position 174 of α_{tr}. An arginine is conserved in an equivalent position in all of the known α-subunits (LOCHRIE and SIMON 1988; STRATHMANN and SIMON 1990). It is thus very likely, albeit not proven, that this arginine serves as the major ADP-ribose acceptor in other cholera-toxin-sensitive α-subunits as well.

Of the 20 mammalian α-subunits identified to date by molecular cloning (SIMON et al. 1991), seven are sensitive to ADP-ribosylation by pertussis toxin. One additional pertussis toxin substrate with an apparent molecular mass of 43 kDa (and hence termed α_{43}) has been discovered in human erythrocytes and several other tissues (IYENGAR et al. 1987). The protein appears to be closely

Table 1. Pertussis-toxin-sensitive G protein α-subunits

cDNA[a]	M_r[b]	Residues	C-terminal sequence[c]	Electrophoretic behavior of encoded protein[d]		Effector[f]
				SDS-PAGE	SDS/Urea-PAGE[e]	
α_{i1}	40.4	354	KNNLKDCGLF	41	42	Adenylyl cyclase (↓)[g]
α_{i2}	40.5	355	KNNLKDCGLF	40	40	Phospholipase C (↑)[g]
α_{i3}	40.4	354	KNNLKECGLY	41	41	Phospholipase D (↑)[g]
						Phospholipase A_2 (↑)[g,h]
						K^+ channels (↑)[g]
						Ca^{2+} channels (↑)[g]
α_{43}	?	?	?	43	44	?
α_{o1}[i]	40.1	354	ANNLRGCGLY	39	40[j]	Ca^{2+} channels (↓)[k]
α_{o2}[i]	40.1	354	AKNLRGCGLF	39	39[j]	K^+ channels (↑)[k]
						Phospholipase C (↑)[k]
α_{t1}	40.0	350	KGNLKDCGLF[l]	39	?	Retinal cGMP PDE (rods) (↑)
α_{t2}	40.1	354	KENLKDCGLF	41[m]	?	Retinal cGMP PDE (cones)(↑)[m]

[a] See LOCHRIE and SIMON 1988 for references
[b] Predicted relative molecular mass $\times 10^{-3}$
[c] The cysteine residue ADP-ribosylated by pertussis toxin is underlined
[d] Apparent relative molecular mass $\times 10^{-3}$
[e] See Fig. 1 and GIERSCHIK et al. 1989
[f] See BIRNBAUMER 1990, and GIERSCHIK et al. 1990b for references
[g] Relevant α_i subtype(s) unknown
[h] CANTIELLO et al. 1990
[i] HSU et al. 1990, STRATHMANN et al. 1990, TSUKAMOTO et al. 1991
[j] SPICHER et al. 1991a, 1991b
[k] Relevant α_0 subtype(s) unknown
[l] Human sequence see LEREA et al. 1989
[m] See LEREA et al. 1989 for further information

related to α_{i3} by immunochemical criteria (CARTY and IYENGAR 1990). The structural properties of the pertussis-toxin-sensitive G protein α-subunits are summarized in Table 1.

6 Molecular Mechanisms of G Protein ADP-Ribosylation by Pertussis Toxin

6.1 ADP-Ribosylation of Retinal Transducin

Although the molecular mechanisms by which pertussis toxin ADP-ribosylates G proteins are very similar or in many respects even identical for all toxin-sensitive G proteins, retinal transducin remains the prototype among the toxin substrates. This is due to the enormous abundance of both rhodopsin and transducin in retinal rod outer segments, which markedly facilitates biochemical studies of both receptor–G protein coupling and G protein modification by bacterial toxins.

The α-subunit of retinal rod transducin is an excellent substrate for ADP-ribosylation by pertussis toxin, both in its native membrane environment and when the purified protein is treated with the toxin in solution (VAN DOP et al. 1984b; WATKINS et al. 1984, 1985). The latter finding demonstrates that ARF-like proteins are not involved in pertussis toxin-mediated ADP-ribosylation of G proteins. The amino acid residue ADP-ribosylated by pertussis toxin in α_{tr} is a cysteine in position 347, which corresponds to the fourth amino acid from the C-terminus (WEST et al. 1985). Thus cholera and pertussis toxin ADP-ribosylate α_{tr} at distinct sites. It is very likely that a cysteine present in position -4 from the C-terminus in all other known pertussis toxin substrates (Table 1) is modified by the toxin in these proteins as well (HSIA et al. 1985; HOSHINO et al. 1990).

The ability of α_{tr} to serve as a pertussis toxin substrate is markedly dependent on the association of the protein with $\beta\gamma_t$ and guanine nucleotides, and on the presence of the light receptor rhodopsin in the ADP-ribosylation mixture. $\beta\gamma$-subunits markedly enhance the ADP-ribosylation of purified α_{tr} (WATKINS et al. 1985) (Fig. 4). Recent evidence suggests that the C-terminal processing of the γ-subunit is essential for the enhancement of α_{tr} ADP-ribosylation by $\beta\gamma_t$ (OHGURO et al. 1990). Whether there is an absolute requirement of $\beta\gamma_t$ for ADP-ribosylation of α_{tr} is uncertain. In two reports, ADP-ribosylation of α_{tr} was only reduced, but not completely abolished in the absence of $\beta\gamma_t$, in particular in the presence of ATP and certain phospholipids (WATKINS et al. 1985; MOSS et al. 1986). Whether this "basal" ADP-ribosylation of α_{tr} was due to the presence of $\beta\gamma_t$ contaminating the α_{tr} preparations remains to be examined. Note that $\beta\gamma$-subunits have been reported to catalytically support the ADP-ribosylation of α-subunits by pertussis toxin (CASEY et al. 1989). Thus, a minute quantity of $\beta\gamma_t$ could have enhanced the radiolabeling of "pure" α_{tr} in the above studies.

In native rod outer segments, ADP-ribosylation of transducin was reported to be reduced by about 95% when bleached, rather than dark-adapted membranes were used in the absence of exogeneous guanine nucleotides (VAN DOP et al. 1984b). This interesting observation was taken by the authors to suggest that the receptor-coupled (i.e., guanine nucleotide-free) form of transducin is not a pertussis toxin substrate (possibly because the ADP-ribosylation site on α_{tr} is masked by the activated receptor; see Fig. 4). Interestingly, guanosine-5′-(2-0-thio)diphosphate (GDP[S]) markedly stimulated the ADP-ribosylation of α_{tr} complexed by light-activated rhodopsin, suggesting that binding of guanine nucleoside diphosphates to the G protein relaxes—at least to some extent—the receptor–G protein interaction, which would then lead to an exposure of the ADP-ribosylation site to the toxin (VAN DOP et al. 1984b) (Fig. 3). Although this concept is very attractive, it is important to note that in two subsequent studies, the investigators failed to see in inhibition of pertussis toxin-mediated ADP-ribosylation by photolyzed rhodopsin (WATKINS et al. 1984, 1985). The reason(s) for these discrepancies are not entirely clear, however, in one study (WATKINS et al. 1985), ADP-ribosylation of transducin was examined in a reconstituted system using a molar ratio of bleached rhodopsin to transducin that was by far lower ($\approx$ 0.6:1) than the ratio present in native rod outer segments ($\approx$ 10:1; KÜHN 1981). Thus, the amount of receptor used in this study was probably too low to observe the effects seen by VAN DOP et al. (1984b). In the other study (WATKINS et al. 1984), where ADP-ribosylation of transducin was analyzed in native rod outer segments, the reaction was performed at a higher toxin concentration and for a much longer time (3.5 h vs. 30 min used by VAN DOP and colleagues). It is important to keep in mind in this context that the effect of a particular agent on G protein ADP-ribosylation may be overlooked if only single point measurements are obtained. Clearly, more detailed studies of the time course of the modification are necessary in these cases (see MATTERA et al. 1986, for a detailed discussion of this issue).

6.2 ADP-Ribosylation of G_i/G_o-Like G Proteins

The molecular mechanisms involved in pertussis toxin-mediated ADP-ribosylation of G proteins of the G_i/G_o subfamily are very similar to those observed with retinal transducin. This is particularly true when the G protein ADP-ribosylation is studied following the reconstitution of the G protein with a receptor protein, as done by TSAI et al. (1984), who reconstituted partially purified rabbit liver α_i and $\beta\gamma$-subunits with retinal rhodopsin (TSAI et al. 1984). Retinal rhodopsin is capable of replacing inhibitory receptors of adenylyl cylase in reconstituted systems, as it is fully capable of interacting with and activating G_i (KANAHO et al. 1984; CERIONE et al. 1985). As observed with α_{tr} (see above), $\beta\gamma$-subunits markedly enhanced ADP-ribosylation of α_i. This effect was particularly prominent in the absence of ATP. Interestingly, photolyzed rhodopsin markedly inhibited the ADP-ribosylation of the G_i holoprotein in the absence of guanine nucleotides, which is very reminiscent of the effects observed by VAN DOP et al. (1984b) for retinal transducin. Note that in this study rhodopsin was present in marked molar excess of G_i ($\approx 40:1$), i.e., at a concentration sufficiently high to complex a significant quantity of G_i. In the presence of photolyzed rhodopsin, the addition of a variety of guanine nucleotides markedly enhanced ADP-ribosylation of G_i. Maximal stimulation was observed with GDP, GDP[S], and GTP. Surprisingly, the GTP analog guanosine-5'-(α,β-methylene)triphosphate (Gpp(CH_2p), GppNHp, and guanosine-5'-(3-*O*-thio)-triphosphate GTP[S] also stimulated ADP-ribosylation, albeit to a lesser extent than the other guanine nucleotides (see below).

Similar to transducin, purified G_i and G_o proteins are excellent substrates for pertussis toxin, even in the absence of any additional protein factor and a lipid bilayer. All variants of α_i and α_o so far examined require $\beta\gamma$-subunits in order to be ADP-ribosylated by pertussis toxin (NEER et al. 1984; HUFF and NEER 1986; KATADA et al. 1986a; GIERSCHIK et al. 1987; CASEY et al. 1989) (Fig. 5). This requirement also holds true for recombinant α_i- and α_o-subunits produced in *E. coli*, in reticulocyte lysates by in vitro translation, or in mammalian cells by DNA transfection (LINDER et al. 1990; HSU et al. 1990; JONES et al. 1990). When the α-subunits were expressed in *E. coli* less that 2% of the protein that could be modified in the presence of $\beta\gamma$-subunits was ADP-ribosylated in its absence (LINDER et al. 1990).

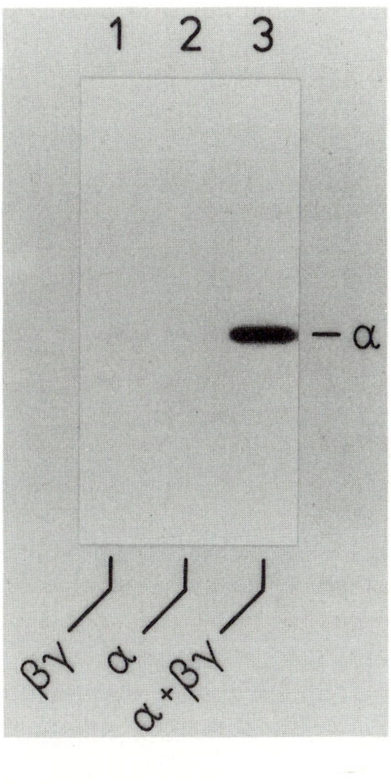

Fig. 5. Requirement of $\beta\gamma$-subunits for ADP-ribosylation of purified α_{i2} by pertussis toxin. $\beta\gamma$-subunits purified from bovine rod outer segments and α_{i2} purified from bovine neutrophils were treated alone (*lanes 1* and *2*) or in combination (*lane 3*) with dithiothreitol-activated pertussis toxin and [^{32}P]NAD$^+$. Subsequently, the samples were subjected to SDS-PAGE and autoradiography was performed. The position of the [^{32}P]ADP-ribosylated α_{i2} is indicated on the *right* (see GIERSCHIK et al. 1987, for further information)

The precise mechanism(s) by which $\beta\gamma$-subunits enhance ADP-ribosylation of pertussis-toxin-sensitive α-subunits are unknown. Protection of α-subunits from denaturation may contribute to a considerable extent. This is because heterotrimeric G proteins may dissociate under certain conditions (e.g., low protein concentration) even in the absence of activating ligands (SMIGEL et al. 1982). The free α-subunit has a considerably lower affinity for GDP than the heterotrimeric protein and is thus more likely to lose bound GDP (HIGASHIJIMA et al. 1987). Unliganded α-subunits are exceptionally labile and thus rapidly lost by denaturation (SMIGEL et al. 1982; NORTHUP et al. 1983a, b). Addition of $\beta\gamma$-dimers and/or exogeneous guanine nucleotides counteracts subunit dissociation and/or loss of guanine nucleotide and thus markedly enhances the amount of viable α-subunits that are available for toxin modification (KATADA et al. 1986a; MATTERA et al. 1986). A second, possibly even more important mechanism for the stimulatory effect of $\beta\gamma$-subunits on ADP-ribosylation of α-subunits by pertussis toxin is an $\beta\gamma$-dimer-induced conformational change of the GDP-liganded α-subunit that is unrelated to α-subunit stability. This suggestion is based on the observation that $\beta\gamma$-subunits led to a marked ($\approx$10-fold) stimulation of ADP-ribosylation of α_i and α_o, even after care was taken to prevent denaturation of the α-subunits by inclusion of GTP in the incubation mixture (KATADA et al. 1986a).

The effects of guanine nucleotides and Mg^{2+} on pertussis-toxin-mediated ADP-ribosylation of G proteins are complex and, it least in part, still poorly understood. This is mainly due to the fact that both agents probably exert multiple effects in the toxin-catalyzed ADP-ribosylation reaction. For example, magnesium ions have been reported by one group to inhibit activation of the toxin by ATP (MOSS et al. 1986). Another group observed a marked inhibition of the toxin-mediated modification of human erythrocyte G_i by Mg^{2+}, Mn^{2+}, and Ca^{2+}, but was unable to observe an effect of Mg^{2+} on the ability of ATP to activate the toxin (MATTERA et al. 1986). Interestingly, Mg^{2+} was a particuarly potent inhibitor when guanine nucleotides were absent from the incubation medium. This observation, together with the previous finding by the same group that Mg^{2+} promoted aggregation of purified G_s (CODINA et al. 1984), led the authors to suggest that Mg^{2+} may inhibit formation of ADP-ribosyl-G_i by causing denaturation of the protein (MATTERA et al. 1986). Note that millimolar concentrations of Mg^{2+} have been suggested to promote the release of GDP from heterotrimeric G proteins (HIGASHIJIMA et al. 1987), a process that likely renders the protein more susceptible to denaturation.

Similar to Mg^{2+}, guanine nucleotides, which are either added on purpose or unintentionally added as a contaminant with the ATP used to activate the toxin, affect G protein ADP-ribosylation by acting at several levels. First, GTP, GDP, GDP[S], and even GTP[S] have been reported to interact directly with and facilitate the activation of pertussis toxin just like ATP (or AppNHp) (MATTERA et al. 1986, 1987). This effect was particularly prominent when ATP was absent from the incubation medium. Second, as already discussed, guanine nucleotides may act as G protein stabilizers and thereby enhance

ADP-ribosylation (MATTERA et al. 1986; KATADA et al. 1986a). Third, binding of stable GTP analogs such as GTP[S] to the G protein induces a conformation that is only poorly or not at all ADP-ribosylated by the toxin (BOKOCH et al. 1984; HUFF and NEER 1986; NAVON and FUNG 1987; MATTERA et al. 1987; JONES et al. 1990). Interestingly, subunit dissociation does not appear to be required for GTP[S]-mediated inhibition of G_i-ADP-ribosylation (MATTERA et al. 1987). Finally, as suggested above, both guanosine nucleoside di- and triphosphates as well as their analogs may loosen the interaction of the G protein with an activated receptor and thus expose the ADP-ribosylation site (VAN DOP et al. 1984b; TSAI et al. 1984). Only if one considers each one of these actions is one able to rationalize some of the seemingly paradoxical effects of guanine nucleotides on pertussis-toxin-mediated G protein ADP-ribosylation. For example, the observation that poorly hydrolyzable GTP analogs stimulated ADP-ribosylation of G_i when reconstituted with photolyzed rhodopsin (TSAI et al. 1984) is certainly rather puzzling in light of the fact that these nucleotides are inhibitory in most other cases. However, as shown schematically for GTP in Fig. 4, binding of these analogs to a receptor-bound G-protein is well known to disrupt the receptor–G protein interaction, which could easily give rise, albeit only transiently, to a G protein that is a better substrate for the toxin than the one complexed to the receptor.

A very important question concerning the molecular mechanisms of pertussis-toxin-mediated ADP-ribosylation of G proteins is which of the structural elements of a given α-subunit (aside from the cystein in position -4 from the C-terminus) are absolutely required for the toxin-mediated modification. Although this question is still subject to further investigation, several initial conclusions can already be drawn from the literature. First, it is clear that the $\approx$20 amino terminal residues of the α-subunit are absolutely required for pertussis-toxin-mediated ADP-ribosylation (WATKINS et al. 1985; NAVON and FUNG 1987; NEER et al. 1988). As the same region is also required for the association of the α-subunit with $\beta\gamma$-dimers (NAVON and FUNG 1987; NEER et al. 1988), it is very likely that an amino terminal truncation precludes the ADP-ribosylation of α-subunits by preventing the formation of the $\alpha\beta\gamma$-heterotrimer. Modification of the N-terminal residue by myristoylation does not appear to be an absolute requirement for ADP-ribosylation (JONES et al. 1990). Note, however, that N-terminal myristoylation markedly reduces the amount of $\beta\gamma$ necessary to support ADP-ribosylation of recombinant α_{o1} (LINDER et al. 1991).

Integrity of the α-subunit C-terminus is important for ADP-ribosylation by pertussis toxin. This is based on the observation that treatment of α_o with carboxypeptides A, which is expected to remove the two carboxyl terminal residues, Leu^{353} and Tyr^{354}, but not the substrates amino acid Cys^{351}, prevented ADP-ribosylation of α_o (NEER et al. 1988). The ability of the protein to interact with $\beta\gamma$ appeared to be unaltered by this treatment. Similar results were reported recently from the laboratory of Moss and Vaughan (TSUCHIYA et al. 1990; AVIGAN et al. 1991) for the ADP-ribosylation of recombinant α_{o1} mutant proteins by pertussis toxin.

In essence, deletion of two C-terminal residues or replacement of the penultimate Leu^{353} by Gly or Ala, or of Gly^{352} by Asp abolished ADP-ribosylation. In contrast, deletion of Tyr^{354} resulted in a protein that was still ADP-ribosylated by the toxin (see AVIGAN et al. 1991 for further information). Also pertinent to this issue, replacement of the tripeptide Gln^{390}-Tyr^{391}-Glu^{392} of α_{s1} (394 residues) by Asp^{390}-Cys^{391}-Gly^{392} (a sequence corresponding to that found in all three forms of α_i; see Table 1) generated an α-subunit that was only poorly ADP-ribosylated by pertussis toxin, despite the fact that the mutant protein contained a Cys in position -4 from the C-terminus and appeared to interact with the $\beta\gamma$-dimer (FREISSMUTH and GILMAN 1989).

A similar finding was obtained by OSAWA et al. (1990), who showed that replacement of the carboxy terminal 38 residues of α_{s1} by the 36 carboxy terminal residues of α_{i2} did not suffice to make the chimeric protein pertussis-toxin-sensitive. Results presented in the latter study also demonstrated that two amino-terminal domains of α_{i2} are required for ADP-ribosylation of the α_{s1}/α_{i2} fusion protein (in addition to the 36 amino acid α_{i2} carboxyl terminus). One domain is expected to lie between residues 1 through 64, the other between residues 65 through 212. It has been suggested that both domains are necessary for the interaction of α-subunits with the $\beta\gamma$-dimer (OSAWA et al. 1990). Although more experimentation is required do substantiate this hypothesis, the concept is consistent with the earlier observation that sulfhydryl alkylation of Cys^{108} of α_o by *N*-ethylmaleimide blocks ADP-ribosylation of the protein (WINSLOW et al. 1987), presumably by preventing the association of α_o with $\beta\gamma$-subunits (HOSHINO et al. 1990).

7 Functional Consequences of G Protein ADP-Ribosylation Pertussis Toxin

The main functional consequence of pertussis-toxin-mediated G protein ADP-ribosylation is an uncoupling of the receptor from effector regulation. The number of transmembrane signaling systems affected by pertussis toxin in this way is considerable and still increasing. It includes the pathways leading to inhibition of adenylyl cyclase, stimulation of phospholipases C, D, and A_2, stimulation of retinal cyclic guanosine monophosphate (cGMP) phosphodiesterase(s), and opening or closing of various ion channels and probably many more (see GIERSCHIK et al. 1990b; BIRNBAUMER et al. 1990, for recent reviews and further references).

The molecular mechanisms leading to the toxin-mediated inhibition of receptor–effector interaction have been analyzed in detail using membrane preparations, reconstituted systems consisting of receptors and/or G proteins implanted into artificial lipid bilayers, and purified G proteins in solution. As a result of these studies, it is now generally agreed that ADP-ribosylation by pertussis toxin prevents the interaction of the agonist-activated receptor with the GDP-liganded G protein (Fig. 4). Evidence in support of this concept is threefold. First, G protein ADP-ribosylation prevents formation of a receptor-G protein complex that binds agonists with high affinity. This phenomenon has been demonstrated in many membrane systems as well as in phospholipid vesicles (see MOSS and VAUGHAN 1988, for references). Second, pertussis toxin treatment of hamster adipocyte membranes led to a marked decrease in the α_2-adrenoceptor-mediated release of [^{3}H]GDP from membrane bound G_i (which had been prelabeled with [^{3}H]GTP prior to the release assay) (MURAYAMA and UI 1984). Third, retinal transducin ADP-ribosylated by pertussis toxin bound less tightly to photolyzed rhodopsin than did the unmodified G protein. Thus, ADP-ribosylated transducin detached from rod outer segment membranes even at physiologic ionic strength and in the absence of guanine nucleotides (VAN DOP et al. 1984b). It is important to note that none of the "intrinsic" G protein functions (i.e., GDP release, GTP[S] binding, GTPase activity, and subunit dissociation) were altered when purified G_i proteins were examined that had been treated with pertussis toxin (HAGA et al. 1985; ENOMOTO and ASAKAWA 1986; HUFF and NEER 1986; KATADA et al. 1986b; SUNYER et al. 1989; CASEY et al. 1989). Furthermore, pertussis toxin did not affect inhibition of cyclic adenosine monophosphate (cAMP) accumulation by a constitutively active (i.e., receptor-independent) α_{i2} mutant, which was nonetheless a good substrate for pertussis-toxin-mediated ADP-ribosylation (WONG et al. 1990). Thus, there is strong evidence that the major consequence of the toxin-mediated modification is in fact a reduced ability of the G protein to interact with the receptor.

Despite the compelling nature of the concept just developed, there are certain findings in the literature that are not easily explained by it. First, treatment of S49 cyc$^-$ lymphoma cells with pertussis toxin blocked inhibition of adenylyl cyclase by GTP even in the absence of inhibitory hormones (HILDEBRANDT et al. 1983), and markedly increased the time required to observe maximal adenylyl cyclase inhibition by GTP[S] (JAKOBS et al. 1984). Second, pertussis toxin treatment of hamster fibroblasts markedly reduced the stimulation of inositol phosphate production by AlF_4^- (PARIS and POUYSSEGUR et al. 1987). These findings are rather puzzling since inhibition of adenylyl cyclase by GTP or GTP[S] and stimulation of phospholipase C by AlF_4^- (in the absence of a hormonal stimulus) are generally believed to be receptor-independent processes, which should neither be inhibited nor delayed by ADP-ribosylation of G_i. Also pertinent to this issue, pertussis toxin treatment of HL-60 cells markedly reduced basal GTPase activity by and basal [^{35}S]GTP[S] binding to their membranes (GIERSCHIK et al. 1989b, 1991). Note that both activities were assayed in the absence of a receptor-agonist and are thus expected to be receptor-independent.

There are two possibilities that might explain these findings. First, it is conceivable that inhibition of the receptor–G protein interaction is not the only functional consequence of G protein ADP-ribosylation by pertussis toxin. This possibility may appear unlikely since ADP-ribosylation of purified G proteins by pertussis toxin has no effect on their various functions (see above). However, it is entirely possible that the functions of membrane-bound G proteins differ significantly from those observed in detergent-containing solutions or even in synthetic lipid vesicles (cf. ASANO and ROSS 1984; FLORIO and STERNWEIS 1985). The second possibility is that unoccupied receptors are not completely silent with regard to G protein activation. This concept has recently gained considerable support from several laboratories, which can be summarized as follows:

1. Reconstitution of the purified β-adrenoceptor into lipid vesicles containing purified G_s significantly enhances GTPase activity of G_s, even in the absence of adrenoceptor agonists (CERIONE et al. 1984).
2. It has been suggested that activation of G proteins by GTP, as opposed to the nonhydrolyzable analogs GppNHp or GTP[S], does not proceed in the absence of a receptor protein, and activation of G proteins by GTP alone may not be receptor-independent but dependent on unoccupied, but nevertheless active receptors (SUNYER et al. 1989).
3. Recent evidence suggests that opioid receptors present in membranes of NG108-15 cells spontaneously associate with G proteins and give rise to increased GTPase activity even in the absence of receptor agonists (COSTA et al. 1990). Interestingly, the increased "basal" GTPase activity is inhibited by certain antagonists (negative antagonists) in a stereospecific fashion (COSTA and HERZ 1989). In contrast to what is known for opioid agonists, the affinity of negative antagonists for opioid receptors is enhanced when G proteins have been ADP-ribosylated by pertussis toxin.

8 Perspectives

Despite the tremendous recent progress in analyzing the structure of pertussis toxin and the molecular mechanisms of pertussis-toxin-mediated G protein ADP-ribosylation, there are a considerable number of questions that remain to be addressed by future experimentation. For example, the physical interaction of the S1 subunit with the G protein substrate is still poorly understood. Likewise, it is not clear whether inhibition of receptor–G protein interaction is in fact the only functional consequence of G protein ADP-ribosylation. Another important line of future investigation will be to analyze which of the structural elements of the various G protein subunits are required for toxin-mediated ADP-ribosylation. Results obtained in these studies will provide important insights into the organisation of α-, β-, and γ-subunits into functional domains. Finally, it will be important to find out whether eukaryocytes contain endogeneous ADP-ribosyltransferases capable of ADP-ribosylating G proteins just like their prokaryotic counterparts. Evidence in support of this concept is emerging (TANUMA et al. 1988; JACOBSON et al. 1990).

References

Ad Hoc Group for the Study of Pertusis Vaccines (1988) Placebo-controlled trial of two acellular pertussis vaccines in Sweden: protective efficacy and adverse effects. Lancet i: 955–960

Antoine R, Locht C (1990) Roles of the disulfide bond and the carboxy-terminal region of the S1 subunit in the assembly and biosynthesis of pertusis toxin. Infect Immun 58: 1518–1526

Asano T, Ross EM (1984) Catecholamine-stimulated guanosine 5′-*O*-(3-thiotriphosphate) binding to the stimulatory GTP-binding protein of adenylate cyclase: kinetic analysis in reconstituted phospholipid vesicles. Biochemistry 23: 5467–5471

Askelöf P, Rodmalm K, Wrangsell G, Larsson U, Svenson SB, Cowell JL, Unden A, Bartfai T (1990) Pertussis toxin-catalyzed ADP-ribosylation of guanine nucleotide-binding proteins: effects of in vitro mutagenesis at the carboxyterminus of $G_{0\alpha}$. FASEB J 5: A4041 (Abstract)

Avigan J, Murthag JJ Jr, Stevens LA, Angus CW, Moss J, Vaughan M (1991) Requirements for pertussis toxin-catalyzed ADP-ribosylation of guanine nucleotide-binding proteins: effects of in vitro mutagenesis at the carboxyterminus of $G_{0\alpha}$. FASEB J 5: A4041 (Abstract)

Backlund PS, Simonds WF, Spiegel AM (1990) Carboxymethylation and COOH-terminal processing of the brain G protein γ-subunit. J Biol Chem 265: 15572–15576

Barbieri JT, Cortina G (1988) ADP-ribosyltransferase mutations in the catalytic S-1 subunit of pertussis toxin. Infect Immun 56: 1934–1941

Barbieri JT, Mende-Mueller LM, Rappuoli R, Collier RJ (1989a) Photolabelling of Glu-129 of the S-1 subunit of pertussis toxin with NAD. Infect Immun 57: 3549–3554

Barbieri JT, Moloney BK, Mende-Mueller LM (1989b) Expression and secretion of the S-1 subunit and C180 peptide of pertussis toxin in *Escherichia coli*. Infect Immun 171: 4362–4369

Barinaga M (1991) How the nose knows: olfactory receptors cloned. The abundant variety of receptors has powerful implications for the brain's processing of smells. Science 252: 209–210

Bartoloni A, Pizza M, Bigio M, Nucci D, Ashwort LA, Irons LI, Robinson A, Burns D, Manclark C, Sato H, Rappuoli R (1988) Mapping of a protective epitope of pertussis toxin by in vitro refolding of recombinant fragments. Bio/Technology 6: 709–712

Bertrand P, Sanford J, Rudolph U, Codina J, Birnbaumer L (1990) At least three alternatively spliced mRNAs encoding two α subunits of the G_o GTP-binding protein can be expressed in a single tissue. J Biol Chem 265: 18576–18580

Birnbaumer L (1990) G proteins in signal transduction. Ann Rev Pharmacol Toxicol 30: 675–705

Birnbaumer L, Abramowitz J, Brown AM (1990) Receptor-effector coupling by G proteins. Biochim Biophys Acta 1031: 163–224

Black WJ, Munoz JJ, Peacock MG, Schad PA, Cowell JL, Burchall JJ, Lim M, Kent A, Steinman L, Falkow S (1988) ADP-ribosyltransferase activity of pertussis toxin and immunomodulation by *Bordella pertussis*. Science 240: 656–659

Bokoch GM, Katada T, Northup JK, Ui M, Gilman AG (1984) Purification and properties of the inhibitory guanine nucleotide-binding regulatory component of adenylate cyclase. J Biol Chem 259: 3560–3567

Bray P, Carter A, Simons C, Guo V, Puckett C, Kamholz J, Spiegel A, Nirenberg M (1986) Human cDNA clones for four species of $G\alpha_s$ signal transduction protein. Proc Natl Acad Sci USA 83: 8893–8897

Brennan MJ, David JL, Kenimer JG, Manclark CR (1988) Lectin-like binding of pertussis toxin to a 165-kilodalton chinese hamster ovary cell glycoprotein. J Biol Chem 263: 4895–4899

Burnette WN, Cieplak W, Mar VL, Kaljot KT, Sato H, Keith JM (1988) Pertussis toxin S1 mutant with reduced enzyme activity and a conserved protective epitope. Science 242: 72–74

Burns DL, Hausman SZ, Lindner W, Robey FA, Manclark CR (1987) Structural characterization of pertussis toxin A subunit. J Biol Chem 262: 17677–17682

Burns DL, Hausman SZ, Witvliet MH, Brennan MJ, Poolman JT, Manclark CR (1988) Biochemical properties of pertussis toxin. Tok J Exp Clin Med 13: 181–185

Burns DL, Manclark CR, Hausman SZ (1990) Pertussis toxin and its mode of entry into eukaryotic cells. In: Manclark CR (ed) Proceedings of the Sixth International Symposium on Pertussis, Department of Health and Human Services, Bethesda, Maryland, DHHS Publication No. (FDA) 90–1164, pp 53–56

Burns DL, Manclark CR (1986) Adenine nucleotide promote dissociation of pertussis toxin subunits. J Biol Chem 261: 4324–4327

Burns DL, Manclark CR (1989) Role of cysteine 41 of the A subunit of pertussis toxin. J Biol Chem 264: 564–568

Buss JE, Mumby S, Casey PJ, Gilman AG, Sefton BM (1987) Myristoylated α subunits of guanine nucleotide-binding regulatory proteins. Proc Natl Acad Sci USA 84: 7493–7497

Cantiello HF, Patenaude CR, Codina J, Birnbaumer L, Ausiello DA (1990) $G_{\alpha i-3}$ regulates epithelial Na^+ channels by activation of phospholipase A_2 and lipoxygenase pathways. J Biol Chem 265: 21624–21628

Capiau C, Petre J, Van Damme J, Puype M, Vandekerkhove J (1986) Protein-chemical analysis of pertussis toxin reveals homology between the subunits S_2 and S_3, between $S_1$and the A chains of enterotoxins of *Vibrio cholerae* and *Escherichia coli* and identifies S_2 as the haptoglobin-binding subunit. FEBS Lett 204: 336–340

Carroll SF, McCloskey JA, Crain PF, Oppenheimer NJ, Marschner TM, Collier RJ (1985) Photoaffinity labeling of diphtheria toxin fragment A with NAD: structure of the photoproduct at position 148. Proc Natl Acad Sci USA 82: 7237–7241

Carroll SF, Collier RJ (1987) Active site of *Pseudomonas areuginosa* exotoxin A: glumatic acid 553 is photolabeled by NAD and shows functional homology with glutamic acid 148 of diphtheria toxin. J Biol Chem 262: 8707–8711

Carty DJ, Iyengar R (1990) A 43 kDA form of the GTP-binding protein G_{i3} in human erythrocytes. FEBS Lett 262: 101–103

Casey PJ, Graziano MP, Gilman AG (1989) G protein $\beta\gamma$ subunits from bovine brain and retina: equivalent catalytic support of ADP-ribosylation of α subunits by pertussis toxin but differential interactions with $G_s\alpha$. Biochemistry 28: 611–616

Cassel D, Selinger Z (1977) Mechanism of adenylate cyclase activation by cholera toxin: inhibition of GTP hydrolysis at the regulatory site. Proc Natl Acad Sci USA 74: 3307–3311

Cassel D, Levkovitz H, Selinger Z (9177) The regulatory GTPase cyclase of turkey erythrocyte adenylate cyclase. J Cyclic Nucleotide Res 3: 393–406

Cerione RA, Codina J, Benovic JL, Lefkowitz RJ, Birnbaumer L, Caron MG (1984) The mammalian β_2-adrenergic receptor: reconstitution of functional interactions between pure receptor and pure stimulatory nucleotide binding protein of the adenylate cyclase system. Biochemistry 23: 4519–4525

Cerione RA, Staniszewski C, Benovic JL, Lefkowitz RJ, Caron MG, Gierschik P, Somers RL, Spiegel AM, Codina J, Birnbaumer L (1985) Specificity of the functional interactions of the β-adrenergic receptor and rhodopsin with guanine nucleotide regulatory proteins reconstituted in phospholipid vesicles. J Biol Chem 260: 1493–1500

Cieplak W, Locht C, Mar VL, Burnette WN, Keith JM (1990) Photolabelling of mutant forms of the S1 subunit of pertussis toxin with NAD^+. Biochem J 268: 547–551

Cockle SA (1989) Identification of an active-site residue in subunit S1 of pertussis toxin by photocrosslinking to NAD. FEBS Lett 249: 329–332

Codina J, Hildebrandt JD, Brinbaumer L, Sekura RD (1984) Effects of guanine nucleotides and Mg on human erythrocyte N_i and N_s, the regulatory components of adenylyl cyclase. J Biol Chem 259: 11408–11418

Cody CL, Baraff LJ, Cherry JD, March SM, Manclark CR (1981) Nature and rates of adverse reactions associated with DTP and DT immunizations in infants and in children. Pediatrics 68: 650–660

Cortina G, Barbieri JT (1989) Role of tryptophan 26 in the NAD glycohydrolase reaction of the S-1 subunit of pertussis toxin. J Biol Chem 264: 17322–17328

Cortina G, Barbieri JT (1991) Localization of a region of the S1 subunit of pertussis toxin required for efficient ADP-ribosyltransferase activity. J Biol Chem 266: 3022–3030

Costa T, Herz A (1989) Antagonists with negative intrinsic activity at δ opioid receptors coupled to GTP-binding proteins. Proc Natl Acad Sci USA 86: 7321–7325

Costa T, Lang J, Gless C, Herz A (1990) Spontaneous association between opioid receptors and GTP-binding regulatory proteins in native membranes: specific regulation by antagonists and sodium ions. Mol Pharmacol 37: 383–394

De Magistris MT, Romano M, Bartoloni A, Rappuoli R, Tagliabue A (1989) Human T cell clones define S1 subunit as the most immunogenic moiety of pertussis toxin and determine its epitope map. J Exp Med 169: 1519–1532

Domenighini M, Montecucco C, Ripka WC, Rappuoli R (1991) Computer modelling of the NAD binding site of ADP-ribosylating toxins: active-site structure and mechanism of NAD binding. Mol Microbiol 5: 23–31

Enomoto K, Asakawa T (1986) Inhibition of catalytic unit of adenylate cyclase and activation of GTPase of N_i protein by $\beta\gamma$-subunits of GTP-binding proteins. FEBS Lett 202: 63–68

Ferguson KM, Higashijima T, Smigel MD, Gilman AG (1986) The influence of bound GDP on the kinetics of guanine nucleotide binding to G proteins. J Biol Chem 261: 7393–7399

Florio VA, Sternweis PC (1985) Reconstitution of resolved muscarinic cholinergic receptors with purified GTP-binding proteins. J Biol Chem 260: 3477–3483

Freissmuth M, Gilman AG (1989) Mutations of $G_s\alpha$ designed to alter the reactivity of the protein with bacterial toxins: substitutions at Arg^{187} result in loss of GTPase activity. J Biol Chem 264: 21907–21914

Fukada Y, Ohguro H, Saito T, Yoshizawa T, Akino T (1989) $\beta\gamma$-subunit of bovine transducin composed of two components with distinctive γ-subunits. J Biol Chem 264: 5937–5943

Fukada Y, Takao T, Ohguro H, Yoshizawa T, Akino T, Shimonishi Y (1990) Farnesylated γ-subunit of photoreceptor G protein indispensable for GTP-binding. Nature 346: 658–660

Fung BK-K, Yamane HK, Ota IM, Clarke S (1990) The γ subunit of brain G-proteins is methyl esterified as a C-terminal cysteine. FEBS Lett 260: 313–317

Gautam N, Northup J, Tamir H, Simon MI (1990) G protein diversity is increased by associations with a variety of γ subunits. Proc Natl Sci USA 87: 7973–7977

Gierschik P, Jakobs KH (1987) Receptor mediated ADP-ribosylation of a phospholipase C-stimulating G protein. FEBS Lett 224: 219–223

Gierschik P, Sidiropoulos D, Spiegel AM, Jakobs KH (1987) Purification and immunochemical characterization of the major pertussis-toxin-sensitive guanine-nucleotide-binding protein of bovine-neutrophil membranes. Eur J Biochem 165: 185–194

Gierschik P, Sidiropoulos D, Jakobs KH (1989a) Two distinct G_i-proteins mediate formyl peptide receptor signal transduction in human leukemia (HL-60) cells. J Biol Chem 264: 21470–21473

Gierschik P, Sidiropoulos D, Steisslinger M, Jakobs KH (1989b) Na^+ regulation of formyl peptide-receptor-mediated signal transduction in HL-60 cells: evidence that the cation prevents activation of the G-protein by unoccupied receptors. Eur J Pharmacol 172: 481–492

Gierschik P, Sidiropoulos D, Dieterich K, Jakobs KH (1990a) Structure and function of signal-transducing heterotrimeric guanosine triphosphate binding proteins. In: Habenicht A (ed) Growth factors, differentiation factors, and cytokines. Springer, Berlin, Heidelberg, New York, pp 395–413

Gierschik P, Sidiropoulos D, Dieterich K, Jakobs KH (1990b) Transmembrane signalling by G_i-proteins. In: Nahorski SR (ed) Transmembrane signalling, intracellular, messengers and implications for drug development. Wiley, Chichester, pp 73–89

Gierschik P, Moghtader R, Straub C, Dieterich K, Jakobs KH (1991) Signal amplification in HL-60 granulocytes: evidence that the chemotactic peptide receptor catalytically activates G-proteins in native plasma membranes. Eur J Biochem 197: 725–732

Gordon JI, Duronio RJ, Rudnick DA, Adams SP, Gokel GW (1991) Protein *N*-myristoylation. J Biol Chem 266: 8647–8650

Haga K, Haga T, Ichiyama A, Katada T, Kurose H, Ui M (1985) Functional reconstitution of purified muscarinic receptors and inhibitory guanine nucleotide regulatory protein. Nature 316: 731–733

Hausman SZ, Manclark CR, Burns DL (1990) Binding of ATP by pertussis toxin and isolated subunits. Biochemistry 29: 6128–6131

Higashijima T, Ferguson KM, Sternweis PC, Smigel MD, Gilman AG (1987) Effects of Mg^{2+} and the $\beta\gamma$-subunit complex on the interactions of guanine nucleotides with G proteins. J Biol Chem 262: 762–766

Hildebrandt JD, Sekura RD, Codina J, Iyengar R, Manclark CR, Birnbaumer L (1983) Stimulation and inhibition of adenylyl cyclase mediated by distinct regulatory proteins. Nature 302: 706–709

Hodges TD, Bailey JC, Fleming JW, Kovacs RJ (1989) Selective parasympathectomy increases the quantity of inhibitory guanine nucleotide-binding proteins in canine cardiac ventricle. Mol Pharmacol 36: 72–77

Hoshino S, Kikkawa S, Takahashi K, Itoh H, Kaziro Y, Kawasaki H, Suzuki K, Katada T, Ui M (1990) Identification of sites for alkylation by *N*-ethylmaleimde and pertussis toxin-catalyzed ADP-ribosylation on GTP-binding proteins. FEBS Lett 276: 227–231

Hsia JA, Tsai S-C, Adamik R, Yost DA, Hewlett EL, Moss J (1985) Amino acid-specific ADP-ribosylation: sensitivity to hydroxylamine of [cysteine(ADP-ribose)] protein and [arginine-(ADP-ribose)] protein linkages. J Biol Chem 260: 16187–16191

Hsu WH, Rudolph U, Sanford J, Bertrand P, Olate J, Nelson C, Moss LG, Boyd III AE, Codina J, Birnbaumer L (1990) Molecualr cloning of a novel splice variant of the α subunit of the mammalian G_o protein. J Biol Chem 265: 11220–11226

Huff RM, Neer EJ (1986) Subunit interactions of native and ADP-ribosylated α_{39} and α_{41}, two guanine nucleotide-binding proteins from bovine cerebral cortex. J Biol Chem 261: 1105–1110

Iiri T, Tohkin M, Morishima N, Ohoka Y, Ui M, Katada T (1989) Chemotactic peptide receptor-supported ADP-ribosylation of a pertussis toxin substrate GTP-binding protein by cholera toxin in neutrophil-type HL-60 cells. J Biol Chem 264: 21394–21400

Iyengar R, Rich KA, Herberg JT, Grenet D, Mumby S, Codina J (1987) Identification of a new GTP-binding protein: a $M_r = 43000$ substrate for pertussis toxin. J Biol Chem 262: 9239–9245

Iyengar R, Rich KA, Herberg JT, Premont RT, Codina J (1988) Glucagon receptor-mediated activation of G_s is accompanied by subunit dissociation. J Biol Chem 263: 15348–15353

Jacobson MK, Loflin PT, Aboul-Ela N, Mingmuang M, Moss J, Jacobson EL (1990) Modification of plasma membrane protein cysteine residues by ADP-ribose in vivo. J Biol Chem 265: 10825–10828

Jakobs KH, Aktories K, Schultz G (1984) Mechanism of pertussis toxin action on the adenylate cyclase system: inhibition of the turn-on reaction of the inhibitory regulatory site. Eur J Biochem 140: 177–181

Jiang M, Pandey S, Tran VT, Fong HKW (1991) Guanine nucleotide-binding regulatory proteins in retinal pigment epithelial cells. Proc Natl Acad Sci USA 88: 3907–3911

Jones DT, Reed RR (1989) G_{olf}: an olfactory-neuron-specific G protein involved in odorant signal transduction. Science 244: 790–795

Jones DT, Masters SB, Bourne HR, Reed RR (1990) Biochemical characterization of three stimulatory GTP-binding proteins: the large and small forms of G_s and the olfactory-specific G-protein G_{of}. J Biol Chem 265: 2671–2676

Jones TLZ, Simonds WF, Merendino JJ Jr, Brann MR, Spiegel AM (1990) Myristoylation of an inhibitory GTP-binding protein α subunit is essential for its membrane attachment. Proc Natl Acad Sci USA 87: 568–572

Kahn RA, Goddard C, Newkirk M (1988) Chemical and immunological characterization of the 21-kDa ADP-ribosylation factor of adenylate cyclase. J Biol Chem 263: 8282–8287

Kanaho T, Tsai S-C, Adamik R, Hewlett EL, Moss J, Vaughan M (1984) Rhodopsin-enhanced GTPase activity of the inhibitory GTP-binding protein of adenylate cyclase. J Biol Chem 259: 7378–7381

Kaslow HR, Lesikar DD (1987) Sulfhydryl-alkylating reagents inactive the NAD glycohydrolyase activity of pertussis toxin. Biochemistry 26: 4397–4402

Kaslow HR, Lim LL, Moss J, Lesikar DD (1987) Structure activity analysis of the activation of pertussis toxin. Biochemistry 26: 123–127

Kaslow HR, Schlotterbeck JD, Mar VL, Burnette WN (1989) Alkylation of cysteine 41, but not cysteine 200, decreases the ADP-ribosyltransferase activity of the S1 subunit of pertussis toxin. J Biol Chem 264: 6386–6390

Katada T, Tamura M, Ui M (1983) The A protomer of islet-activating protein, pertussis toxin, as an active peptide catalyzing ADP-ribosylation of a membrane protein. Arch Biochem Biophys 224: 290–298

Katada T, Oinum M, Ui M (1986a) Two guanine nucleotide-binding proteins in rat brain serving as the specific substrate of islet-activating protein, pertussis toxin: interactions of the α-subunits with $\beta\gamma$-subunits in development of their biological activities. J Biol Chem 261: 8182–8191

Katada T, Oinuma M, Ui M (1986b) Mechanisms for inhibition of the catalytic activity of adenylate cyclase by the guanine nucleotide-binding proteins serving as the substrate of islet-activating protein, pertussis toxin. J Biol Chem 261: 5215–5221

Kim KJ, Burnette WN, Sublett RD, Manclark CR, Kenimer JG (1989) Epitopes on the S1 subunit of pertussis toxin recognized by monoclonal antibodies. Infect Immun 57: 944–950

Klinz F-J, Costa T (1989) Cholera toxin ADP-ribosylates the receptor-coupled form of pertussis toxin-sensitive G proteins. Biochem Biophys Res Commun 165: 554–560

Kühn H (1981) Interactions of rod cell proteins with the disk membrane: influence of light, ionic strength, and nucleotides. Curr Top Membr Transp 15: 171–201

Lai RK, Perez-Sala D, Canada FJ, Rando RR (1990) The γ subunit of transducin is farnesylated. Proc Natl Acad Sci USA 87: 7673–7677

Larea CL, Bunt-Milam AH, Hurley JB (1989) α Transducin is present in blue-, green-, and red-sensitive cone photoreceptors in the human retina. Neuron 3: 367–376

Linder ME, Ewald DA, Miller RJ, Gilman AG (1990) Purification and characterization of $G_o\alpha$ and three types of $G_i\alpha$ after expression in *Escherichia coli*. J Biol Chem 265: 8243–8251

Linder ME, Pang I-H, Durinio RJ, Gordon JI, Sternweis PC, Gilman AG (1991) Lipid modifications of G protein subunits: myristoylation of $G_{o\alpha}$ increases its affinity for $\beta\gamma$. J Biol Chem 266: 4654–4659

Lobban MD, Van Heyningen S (1988) Thiol reagents are substrates for the ADP-ribosyltransferase activity of pertussis toxin. FEBS Lett 233: 229–232

Lochrie MA, Simon MI (1988) G protein multiplicity in eukaryotic signal transduction systems. Biochemistry 27: 4957–4965

Locht C, Keith JM (1986) Pertussis toxin gene: nucleotide sequence and genetic organization. Science 232: 1258–1264

Locht C, Barstad PA, Coligan JE, Mayer L, Munoz JJ, Smith SG, Keith JM (1986) Molecular cloning of pertussis toxin genes. Nucl Acid Res 14: 3251–3261

Locht C, Capiau C, Feron C (1989) Identification of amino acid residues essential for the enzymatic activities of pertussis toxin. Proc Natl Acad Sci USA 86: 3075–3079

Locht C, Lobet Y, Feron C, Cieplak W, Keith JM (1990) The role of cysteine 41 in the enzymatic activities of the pertussis toxin S1 subunit as investigated by site-directed mutagenesis. J Biol Chem 265: 4552–4559

Locht C, Cabezon T (1990) Molecular biological studies on the structure-function relationship of pertussis toxin and filamentous hemagglutinin. In: Manclark CR (ed) Proceedings of the Sixth International Symposium on Pertussis, Department of Health and Human Services, Bethesda, Maryland, DHHS Publication No. (FDA) 90–1164, pp 41–52

Maltese WA (1990) Posttranslational modification of proteins by isoprenoids in mammalian cells. FASEB J 4: 3319–3328

Manclark CR (ed) (1990) Proceedings of the Sixth International Symposium on Pertussis, Department of Health and Human Services, United States Public Health Service, Bethesda, Maryland, DHHS Publication No. (FDA) 90–1164, 1990, pp 1–408.

Mattera R, Codina J, Sekura RD, Birnbaumer L (1986) The interaction of nucleotides with pertussis toxin: direct evidence for a nucleotide binding site on the toxin regulating the rate of ADP-ribosylation of N_i, the inhibitory regulatory component of adenylyl cyclase. J Biol Chem 261: 11173–11179

Mattera R, Codina J, Sekura RD, Birnbaumer L (1987) Guanosine 5′-*O*-(3-thiotriphosphate) reduces ADP-ribosylation of the inhibitory guanine nucleotide-binding regulatory protein of adenylyl cyclase (N_i) by pertussis toxin without causing dissociation of the subunits of N_i: evidence of existence of heterotrimeric pt^+ and pt^+ conformations of N_i. J Biol Chem 262: 11247–11251

Miller DL, Ross EM, Alderslade R, Bellman MH, Brawson NSB (1981) Pertussis immunization and serious acute neurological illness in children. Br Med J 282: 1595–1599

Milligan G, McKenzie FR (1988) Opioid peptides promote cholera-toxin-catalysed ADP-ribosylation of the inhibitory guanine-nucleotide-binding protein (G_i) in membranes of neuroblastoma x glioma hybrid cells. Biochem J 252: 369–373

Milligan G (1989) Foetal calf serum enhances cholera toxin-catalyzed ADP-ribosylation of the pertussis toxin-sensitive guanine nucleotide binding protein, G_i2, in rat glioma C6BUI cells. Cell Signal 1: 65–74

Milligan G, Carr C, Gould GW, Mullaney I, Lavan BE (1991) Agonist-dependent, cholera toxin-catalyzed ADP-ribosylation of pertussis toxin-sensitive G-proteins following transfection of the α_2-C10 adrenergic receptor into rat 1 fibroblasts: evidence for the direct interaction of a single receptor with two pertussis toxin-sensitive G-proteins, G_i2 and G_i3. J Biol Chem 266: 6447–6455

Moss J, Stanley SJ, Morin JE, Dixon JE (1980) Activation of choleragen by thiol: protein disulfide oxidoreductase. J Biol Chem 255: 11085–11087

Moss J, Stanley SJ, Burns DL, Hsia JA, Yost DA, Myers GA, Hewlett EL (1983) Activation by thiol of the latent NAD glycohydrolase and ADP-ribosyltransferase activities of *Bordetella pertussis* toxin (islet-activating protein). J Biol Chem 158: 11879–11882

Moss J, Stanley SJ, Watkins PA, Burns DL, Manclark CR, Kaslow HR, Hewlett EL (1986) Stimulation of the thiol-dependent ADP-ribosyltransferase and NAD glycohydrolase activities of *Brodetella pertussis* toxin by adenine nucleotides, phospholipids, and detergents. Biochemistry 25: 2720–2725

Moss J, Vaughan M (1988) ADP-ribosylation of guanyl nucleotide-binding regulatory proteins by bacterial toxins. Adv Enzymol 61: 303–379

Mumby S, Heukeroth RO, Gordon JI, Gilman AG (1990a) G protein α-subunit expression, myristoylation, and membrane association in COS cells. Proc Natl Acad Sci USA 87: 728–732

Mumby SM, Casey PJ, Gilman AG, Gutowski S, Sternweis PC (1990b) G protein γ subunits contain a 20-carbon isoprenoid. Proc Natl Acad Sci USA 87: 5873–5877

Murayama T, Ui M (1984) [^{3}H]GDP release from rat and hamster adipocyte membranes independently linked to receptors involved in activation or inhibition of adenylate cyclase. J Biol Chem 259: 761–769

Navon SE, Fung BK-K (1987) Characterization of transducin from bovine retinal rod outer segments: participation of the amino-terminal region of Tα in subunit interaction. J Biol Chem 262: 15746–15751

Neer EJ, Lok JM, Wolf LG (1984) Purification and properties of the inhibitory guanine nucleotide regulatory unit of brain adenylate cyclase. J Biol Chem 259: 14222–14229

Neer EJ, Pulsifer L, Wolf LG (1988) The amino terminus of G-protein α-subunits is required for interaction with $\beta\gamma$. J Biol Chem 263: 8996–9000

Neer EJ, Clapham DE (1990) Structure and function of G-protein $\beta\gamma$ subunit. In: Iyengar R, Birnbaumer L (eds) G proteins. Academic, San Diego, pp 41–61

Nicosia, A, Perugini M, Franzini C, Casagli MC, Borri MG, Almoni M, Neri P, Ratti G, Rappuoli R (1986) Cloning and sequencing of the pertussis toxin genes: operon structure and gene duplication. Proc Natl Acad USA 83: 4631–4635

Northup JK, Sternweis PC, Gilman AG (1983a) The subunits of the stimulatory regulatory component of adenylate cyclase: resolution, activity, and properties of the 35000-Delton (β) subunit. J Biol Chem 258: 11361–11368

Northup JK, Smigel MD, Sternweis PC, Gilman AG (1983b) The subunits of the stimulatory regulatory component of adenylate cyclase: resolution of the activated 45000-dalton (α) subunit. J Biol Chem 258: 11369–11376

Ohguro H, Fukada Y, Yoshizawa T, Saito T, Akino T (1990) A specific $\beta\gamma$-subunit of transducin stimulates ADP-ribosylation of the α-subunit by pertussis toxin. Biochem Biophys Res Commun 167: 1235–1241

Osawa S, Dhanasekaran N, Woon CW, Johnson GL (1990) $G\alpha_i$-$G\alpha_s$ chimeras define the function of α chain domains in control of G protein activation and $\beta\gamma$ subunit complex interaction. Cell 63: 697–706

Paris S, Pouyssegur J (1987) Further evidence for a phospolipase C-coupled G protein in hamster fibroblasts: induction of inositol phosphate formation by fluoroaluminate and vanadate and inhibition by pertussis toxin. J Biol Chem 262: 1970–1976

Pizza M, Bartoloni A, Prugnola A, Silvstri S, Rappuoli R (1988) Subunit S1 of pertussis toxin: mapping of the regions essential for ADP-ribosyltransferase activity. Proc Natl Acad Sci USA 85: 7521–7525

Pizza M, Covacci A, Bartoloni A, Perugini M, Nencioni L, De Magistris MT, Villa L, Nucci D, Manetti R, Bugnoli M, Giovannoni F, Olivieri R, Barbieri JT, Sato H, Rappuoli R (1989) Mutants of pertussis toxin suitable for vaccine development. Science 246: 497–500

Pizza M, Bugnoli M, Manetti R, Covacci A, Rappuoli R (1990) The subunit S1 is important for pertussis toxin secretion. J Biol Chem 265: 17759–17763

Pizza M, Bugnoli M, Pucci P, Siciliano R, Marino G, Rappuoli R (1991) Further analysis of the sequence of the S1 subunit of pertussis toxin. Infect Immun 59: 1177–1179

Raghavan M, Gotto JW, Scott JV, Schutt CE (1991) Preliminary X-ray crystallographic analysis of holotoxin from *Bordetella pertussis*. J Mol Biol 213: 411–414

Ransnäs LA, Insel PA (1988) Subunit dissociation is the mechanism for hormonal activation of the G_s protein in native membranes. J Biol Chem 263: 17239–17242

Ribeiro-Neto FAP, Mattera R, Hildebrandt JD, Codina J, Field JB, Birnbaumer L, Sekura RD (1985) ADP-ribosylation of membrane components by pertussis and cholera toxin. Methods in Enzymology 109: 566–573

Ribeiro-Neto FAP, Mattera R, Grenet D, Sekura RD, Birnbaumer L, Field JB (1987) Adenosine diphosphate ribosylation of G proteins by pertussis and cholera toxin: different requirements for and effects of guanine nucleotides and Mg^{2+}. Mol Endocrinol 1: 472–481

Sato H, Ito A, Chiba J, Sato Y (1984) Monoclonal antibody against pertussis toxin: effect on toxin activity and pertussis infections. Infect Immun 46: 422–428

Sato H, Sato Y, Ito A, Ohishi I (1987) Effect of monoclonal antibody to pertussis toxin on toxin activity. Infect Immun 55: 909–915

Schultz AM, Tsai S-C, Kung H-F, Oroszlan S, Moss J, Vaughan M (1987) Hydroxylamine-stable covalent linkage of myristic acid in $G_o\alpha$, a guanine nucleotide-binding protein of bovine brain. Biochem Biophys Res Commun 146: 1234–1239

Sekura RD, Fish F, Manclark CR, Meade B (1983) Pertussis toxin: affinity purification of a new ADP-ribosyltransferase. J Biol Chem 258: 14647–14651

Sekura RD, Moss J, Vaughan M (eds) (1985) Pertussis toxin. Academic, Orlando, pp 1–255

Simon MI, Strathmann M, Gautam N (1991) Diversity of G proteins in signal transduction. Science 252: 802–808

Simonds WF, Butrynski JE, Gautam N, Unson CG, Spiegel AM (1991) G-protein $\beta\gamma$-dimers: membrane targeting requires subunit coexpression and intact γ C-A-A-X domain. J Biol Chem 266: 5363–5366

Sixma TK, Pronk SE, Kalk KH, Wartna ES, Van Zanten BAM, Witholt B, Hol WGJ (1991) Crystal structure of a cholera toxin-related heat-labile enterotoxin from *E. coli.* Nature 351: 371–377

Smigel MD, Northup JK, Gilman AG (1982) Characteristics of the guanine nucleotide-binding regulatory component of adenylate cyclase. Recent Progr Horm Res 38: 601–624

Spicher K, Klinz F-J, Nürnberg B, Tychowiecka I, Rosenthal W (1991a) Peptide antibodies distinguish between subtypes of G_o α-subunits. Naunyn-Schmiedeberg's Arch Pharmacol 343: R37 (Abstract)

Spicher K, Klinz F-J, Rudolph U, Codina J, Birnbaumer L, Schultz G, Rosenthal W (1991b) Identification of the G protein α-subunit encoded by α_{o2} cDNA as a 39 kDa pertussis toxin substrate. Biochem Biophys Res Commun 175: 473–479

Storsaeter J, Olin P, Renemar B, Lagergard T, Norberg R, Romanus V, Tiru M (1988) Mortality and morbidity from invasive bacterial infections during a clinical trial of acellular pertussis vaccines in Sweden. Pediater Infect Dis J 7: 637–645

Strathmann M, Wilkie TM, Simon MI (1989) Diversity of the G-protein family: sequences from five additional α subunits in the mouse. Proc Natl Acad Sci USA 86: 7407–7409

Strathmann M, Simon MI (1990) G protein diversity: a distinct class of α subunits is present in vertebrates and invertebrastes. Proc Natl Acad Sci USA 87: 9113–9117

Strathmann M, Wilkie TM, Simon MI (1990) Alternative splicing produces transcripts encoding two forms of the α subunit of GTP-binding protein G_o. Proc Natl Acad Sci USA 87: 6477–6481

Sunyer T, Monastirsky B, Codina J, Birnbaumer L (1989) Studies on nucleotide and receptor regulation of G_i proteins: effects of pertussis toxin. Mol Endocrinol 3: 1115–1124

Tamir H, Fawzi AB, Tamir A, Evans T, Northup JK (1991) G-protein $\beta\gamma$-forms: identity of β and diversity of γ-subunits. Biochemistry 30: 3929–3936

Tamura M, Nogimori K, Murai S, Yajima M, Ito K, Katada T, Ui M, Ishii S (1982) Subunit structure of islet-activating protein, pertussis toxin, in conformity with the A–B model. Biochemistry 21: 5516–5522

Tamura M, Nogimori K, Yajima M, Ase K, Ui M (1983) A role of the B-oligomer moiety of islet-activating protein, pertussis toxin, in development of the biological effects on intact cells. J Biol Chem 258: 6756–6761

Tanuma S, Kawashima K, Endo H (1988) Eukaryotic mono(ADP-ribosyl)transferase that ADP-ribosylates GTP-binding regulatory G_i protein. J Biol Chem 263: 5485–5489

Tsuchiya M, Bliziotes MM, Serventi IM, Price SR, Avigan J, Murtagh JJ, Stevens LA, Angus CW, Walker MW, Newman KB, Helpern JL, Tsai SC, Moss J, Vaughan M (1990) Pertussis toxin substrates: characterization of multiple forms of $G_{o\alpha}$ mRNA and the requirements for toxin-catalyzed ADP-ribosylation of $G_{o\alpha}$ and $G_{t\alpha}$. Manclark CR (ed) Proceedings of the Sixth International Symposium on Pertussis, Department of Health and Human Services, Bathesda, Maryland, DHHS Publication No. (FDA) 90–1164, pp 57–65

Tsukamoto T, Toyama R, Itoh H, Matsuoka M, Kaziro Y (1991) Structure of the human gene and two rat cDNAs encoding the α chain of GTP-binding regulatory protein Go: two different mRNAs are generated by alternative splicing. Proc Natl Acad Sci USA 88: 2974–2978

Ui M (1984) Islet-activating protein, pertussis toxin: a probe for functions of the inhibitory guanine nucleotide regulatory component of adenylate cyclase. Trends Pharmacol Sci 5: 277–279

Ui M (1986) Pertussis toxin as a probe of receptor coupling to inositol lipid metabolism. In: Putney JW (ed) Phosphoinositides and receptor mechanisms. Liss, New York, p 163

Van Dop C, Tsubokawa M, Bourne HR, Ramachandran J (1984a) Amino acid sequence of retinal transducin at the site ADP-ribosylated by cholera toxin. J Biol Chem 259: 696–698

Van Dop C, Yamanaka G, Steinberg F, Sekura RD, Manclark CR, Stryer L, Bourne HR (1984b) ADP-ribosylation of transducin by pertussis toxin blocks the light-stimulated hydrolysis of GTP and cGMP in retinal photoreceptors. J Biol Chem 259: 23–26

Watkins PA, Moss J, Burns DL, Hewlett EL, Vaughan M (1984) Inhibition of bovine rod outer segement GTPase by *Bordetella pertussis* toxin. J Biol Chem 259: 1378–1381

Watkins PA, Burns DL, Kanaho Y, Liu T-Y, Hewlett EL, Moss J (1985) ADP-ribosylation of transducin by pertussis toxin. J Biol Chem 260: 13478–13482

West RE Jr, Moss J, Vaughan M, Liu T, Liu T-Y (1985) Pertussis toxin-catalyzed ADP-ribosylation of transducin: cysteine 347 is the ADP-ribose acceptor site. J Biol Chem 260: 14428–14430

Weiss AA, Hewlett EL (1986) Virulence factors of *Bordetella pertussis.* Ann Rev Microbiol 40: 661–686
Winslow JW, Bradley JD, Smith JA, Neer EJ (1987) Reactive sulfhydryl groups of α_{39}, a guanine nucleotide-binding protein from brain: location and function. J Biol Chem 262: 4501–4507
Witvliet MH, Burns DL, Brennan MJ, Poolman JT, Manclark CR (1989) Binding of pertussis toxin to eucaryotic cells and glycoproteins. Infect Immun 57: 3324–3330
Wong YH, Federman A, Pace AM, Zachary I, Evans T, Pouyssegur J, Bourne HR (1991) Mutant α subunits of G_{i2} inhibit cyclic AMP accumulation. Nature 351: 63–65
Yamamoto T, Nakazawa T, Miyata T, Kaji A, Yokata T (1984) Evolution and structure of two ADP-ribosylation enterotoxins, *Escherichia coli* heat-labile toxin and cholera toxin. FEBS Lett 169: 241–246
Yamane HK, Farnsworth CC, Xie H, Howald W, Fung BK-K, Clarke S, Gelb MH, Glomset JA (1990) Brain G protein γ subunits contain an all-*trans*-geranylgeranyl-cysteine methyl ester at their carboxyl termini. Proc Natl Acad Sci 87: 5868–5872

Clostridial Actin-ADP-Ribosylating Toxins

K. AKTORIES, M. WILLE, and I. JUST

1 Introduction

Several ADP-ribosylating toxins, such as cholera toxin, pertussis toxin, diphtheria toxin, and *Pseudomonas aeruginosa* exotoxin A have been the focus of intensive research for many years. Studies on these toxins, which are described in other chapters of this volume, have brought about insights into the pathogenetic mechanisms of diseases related to the toxin-producing bacteria. Furthermore, especially cholera and pertussis toxins, which ADP-ribosylate GTP-binding proteins, have been proved to be excellent instruments for

Institut für Pharmakologie und Toxikologie der Universität des Saarlandes, 6650 Homburg, FRG

elucidation of the physiological functions of their target proteins (for recent reviews see also MOSS and VAUGHAN 1990).

Recently, a novel family of clostridial ADP-ribosylating toxins have been described which modify actin. These toxins transfer the ADP-ribose moiety from NAD onto actin, a modification which largely changes the functional properties of the target protein. A compelling amount of evidence has been presented showing that the ADP-ribosylation of actin is the molecular basis of the cytotoxic effects of these toxins (previous reviews: AKTORIES and WEGNER 1989; AKTORIES 1990). Members of this family of actin-ADP-ribosylating toxins are *Clostridium botulinum* C2 toxin, *C. perfringens* iota toxin, *C. spiroforme* toxin, and an ADP-ribosyltransferase produced by *C. difficile*. The toxins are not only characterized by a common target but also by their common structure: They are all constructed according to the A–B model and consist of a binding component (B) and an enzyme component (A) which possesses ADP-ribosyltransferase activity. Furthermore, in contrast to other bacterial toxins such as cholera toxin (GILL 1977) or pertussis toxin (TAMURA et al. 1982), which are comprised according to the A–B model, the actin-modifying toxins are binary in structure, having two components linked neither by covalent nor by non-covalent bonds. In this chapter the various actin-ADP-ribosylating toxins and the consequences of this modification are described. As *C. botulinum* C2 toxin and *C. perfringens* iota toxin are the best-studied examples of this toxin family, these two toxins are discussed in more detail.

2 Clostridium Botulinum C2 Toxin

2.1 Toxin Production and Purification

C. botulinum C2 toxin is produced by various strains of *C. botulinum type* C and D (EKLUND and POYSKY 1972; OHISHI and OKADA 1986). These clostridia produce also the botulinum neurotoxin C1 or D (EKLUND and POYSKY 1972) and exoenzyme C3 (AKTORIES et al. 1987; RUBIN et al. 1988). Whereas the structural genes of the neurotoxins C1 and D and of exoenzyme C3 are phage-encoded (EKLUND et al. 1971, 1972; POPOFF et al. 1990), it appears that the DNA encoding C2 toxin is chromosomally located. By acridine orange treatment, these clostridia can be freed of their prophages and, consequently, stop the production of neurotoxins and C3 while still producing C2 toxin (EKLUND et al. 1971, 1972; RUBIN et al. 1988). It appears that the synthesis of C2 toxin is closely related to the sporulation phase of the clostridia. The amount of C2 produced by clostridia is much lower in the vegetative phase than during sporulation (NAKAMURA et al. 1978). The components of the binary C2 toxin are always produced in parallel; however, the ratio in the concentrations of component I and II of the toxin produced by various strains of *C. botulinum* type C and D varies considerably between 1:1 and 1:6 (OHISHI and OKADA 1986).

Botulinum C2 toxin is a binary toxin which consists of two nonlinked components (OHISHI et al. 1980a). Component II (C2II) is responsible for the binding of the toxin to the eukaryotic cell surfaces, whereas component I (C2I) possesses the ADP-ribosyltransferase activity. The purification of the binary botulinum C2 toxin was first reported by OHISHI et al. (1980a). They started with the culture supernatant from *C. botulinum* type C strain 92–13 which produces only C2 toxin but no neurotoxins. The toxin was purified by using ammonium sulfate precipitation (58% saturation), acid precipitation (pH 4.5), DEAE Sephadex chromatography, and carboxymethyl-Sephadex chromatography. The latter step separates C2I and C2II. Final purification to apparent homogeneity was achieved by gel filtration of the separated components.

2.2 C2II, the Binding Component

C2II has a molecular mass of about 100 kDA (OHISHI et al. 1980a). Study of several strains of *C. botulinum* has revealed a heterogeneity in C2II, with molecular masses between 95 kDa and 105 kDa (OHISHI and OKADA 1986). C2II is activated by partial proteolysis in the presence of trypsin, whereby an active 74-kDa protein is relased (OHISHI 1987). It appears that the activated component of C2II binds to the cell surface, thereby inducing a binding site for C2I (OHISHI and MIYAKE 1985; SIMPSON 1989). So far it is unknown whether this binding site is directly located on C2II or on the eukaryotic cells. SIMPSON (1989) presented some evidence that the translocation of C2I into the cell is based on receptor-mediated endocytosis. The cellular transport of the toxin is blocked at 4 °C. At this temperature C2II remains at the cell surface, and still binding of the light component occurs. At 37 °C C2II itself is internalized and, thereafter, no longer accessible for attachment of C2I. Furthermore, the putative inhibitors of endocytosis ammonium chloride and methylamine hydrochloride block the internalization of the toxin. OHISHI (1987) reported that C2II possesses hemagglutinating and hemolytic activities. Again, the trypsin-activated fragment was much more potent. OHISHI showed that the activated 74-kDa binding component forms pentamers, with hemagglutinating and hemolytic activity, whereas the trypsinized monomer of about 74 kDa only possesses hemagglutinating properties. Hemagglutination of trypsin-treated human erythrocytes by C2 toxin is inhibited by galactose, *N*-acetylgalactosamine, *L*-fucose, and mannose, but most effectively inhibited by thyroglobulin and bovine salivary mucin (SUGII and KOZAKI 1990). On the other hand, neuraminidase-treated erythrocytes are more strongly hemolysed than intact or trypsin-treated erythrocytes by activated C2II. From these and other findings it has been suggested that C2II binds to a glycoprotein of the erythrocyte membrane (SUGII and KOZAKI 1990).

2.3 C2I, the Enzyme Component

C2I has reportedly a molecular mass of 50 kDa (OHISHI et al. 1980a). In our laboratory, the purification of C2I results in a protein with an M_r of 45000. A similar M_r of 45000 has been reported by POPOFF et al. (1988). SIMPSON (1984) was the first to report that C2I possesses ADP-ribosyltransferase activity. AKTORIES et al. (1986a, b) identified actin as the physiological target of C2 toxin in cell lysates and demonstrated the ADP-ribosylation of purified actin by the toxin. Modification of actin is highly selective. Neither G proteins, which are substrates of cholera or pertussis toxin, nor other cytoskeletal proteins such as tubulin (unpublished observation) are ADP-ribosylated. As known for other bacterial toxins, C2 toxin transfers mono-ADP-ribose onto its target protein. Typically for mono-ADP-ribosylation reactions, the incorporated ADP-ribose moiety is cleaved by *Crotalus adamanteus* phosphodiesterase, which releases AMP from the modified substrate (AKTORIES et al. 1986b). The K_m of the ADP-ribosylation reaction for NAD is 1–5 μM. As is known for other ADP-ribosylating toxins, C2 toxin possesses NAD-glycohydrolase activity and splits nicotinamide into nicotinic acid and ADP-ribose (OHISHI 1986).

Substrate of the toxin is monomeric G-actin (AKTORIES et al. 1986a), but not polymerized F-actin. Therefore, the mycotoxin phalloidin which induces polymerization and stabilization of F-actin (COOPER 1987) inhibits the toxin-induced ADP-ribosylation of actin (AKTORIES et al. 1986b). The small amount of incorporated label which is observed with F-actin is most probably due to partial depolymerization to G-actin.

By direct protein chemistry analysis it has been shown that C2-toxin attaches ADP-ribose at arginine-177 of actin (VANDEKERCKHOVE et al. 1988). This finding explains why the toxin is able to modify homopolyarginine under extreme conditions (SIMPSON et al. 1988). The half-life of the ADP-ribose-actin linkage is about 2 h in the presence of neutral hydroxylamine (AKTORIES et al. 1988). A similar stability has been reported for the ADP-ribose-arginine linkage catalyzed by cholera toxin (HSIA et al. 1985).

In respect of various actin isoforms, the C2 toxin-induced ADP-ribosylation is characterized by a particular substrate specificity. The toxin modifies β- and γ-nonmuscle actin and γ-smooth muscle actin, but not α-actin isoforms including α-skeletal muscle actin, α-cardiac muscle actin, and α-smooth muscle actin (MAUSS et al. 1990). This finding is surprising because arginine-177 is located at the identical position in all isoforms. Moreover, the various actin isoforms are more than 95% homologous (VANDEKERCKHOVE and WEBER 1979). Since γ-smooth muscle actin, which is modified by C2 toxin, and α-smooth muscle actin, which is not a substrate, differ only in the N-terminal region, it has been suggested that this area defines the substrate specifity for ADP-ribosylation by C2 toxin (MAUSS et al. 1990).

3 Functional Consequences of ADP-Ribosylation of Actin

3.1 Inhibition of Actin Polymerization and "Capping Protein" Function of ADP-Ribosylated Actin

ADP-ribosylation causes dramatic changes in the properties of actin. The modification inhibits the ability of actin to polymerize. This was shown by measuring the viscosity of a G-actin solution by the falling ball method (AKTORIES et al. 1986a) and was confirmed by electron microscopic studies (AKTORIES et al. 1986b). Furthermore, it has been shown that the ADP-ribosylated actin inhibits the polymerization of unmodified G-actin onto actin filaments in a manner characteristic of the interaction of a capping protein with actin filaments. Capping proteins bind to the ends of actin filaments, thereby inhibiting the further polymerization of actin (POLLARD and COOPER 1986). Since the interaction of ADP-ribosylated actin with filaments is inhibited in the presence of gelsolin-capped actin filaments it has been proposed that the modified actin interacts only with the "barbed ends" of actin filaments (WEGNER and AKTORIES 1988; WEIGT et al. 1989). Gelsolin itself is a barbed end capping protein, and it blocks polymerization at the fast-growing ends of filaments without affecting the polymerization or depolymerization at the pointed ends of actin filaments (POLLARD and COOPER 1986). The equilibrium constant for binding of ADP-ribosylated actin for the barbed end of F-actin was found to be about $K_a \approx 10^8 M^{-1}$. By capping the barbed end of F-actin, the critical concentration of actin for polymerization increases to values which correspond to the critical actin concentration at the pointed end of actin filaments (WEGNER and AKTORIES 1988).

Recently, the atomic structure of actin in the actin DNase I complex has been analyzed at a resolution of 2.8 Å (KABSCH et al. 1990; Fig. 1). From these data and from the related atomic model of the actin filament (HOLMES et al. 1990) it has been proposed that arginine-177, the ADP-ribose acceptor of actin, lies near the axis between the two-start helix strands which form the actin filament. With ADP-ribose to arginine-177, the formation of the actin filament is hindered by the bulky group. The only position where the ADP-ribose moiety presents no steric hindrance to formation of the filament is the barbed end of the actin filament. Thus these data agree nicely with the observation that actin acts as barbed end capping protein.

3.2 Inhibition of Actin ATPase Activity

ADP-ribosylation of actin increases the rate of ATP exchange about two fold and inhibits actin-associated ATPase activity (GEIPEL et al. 1989). Several findings indicate that the latter effect is not only the consequence of the inhibition of actin polymerization. First, even at concentrations of Mg^{2+} which are too low to allow

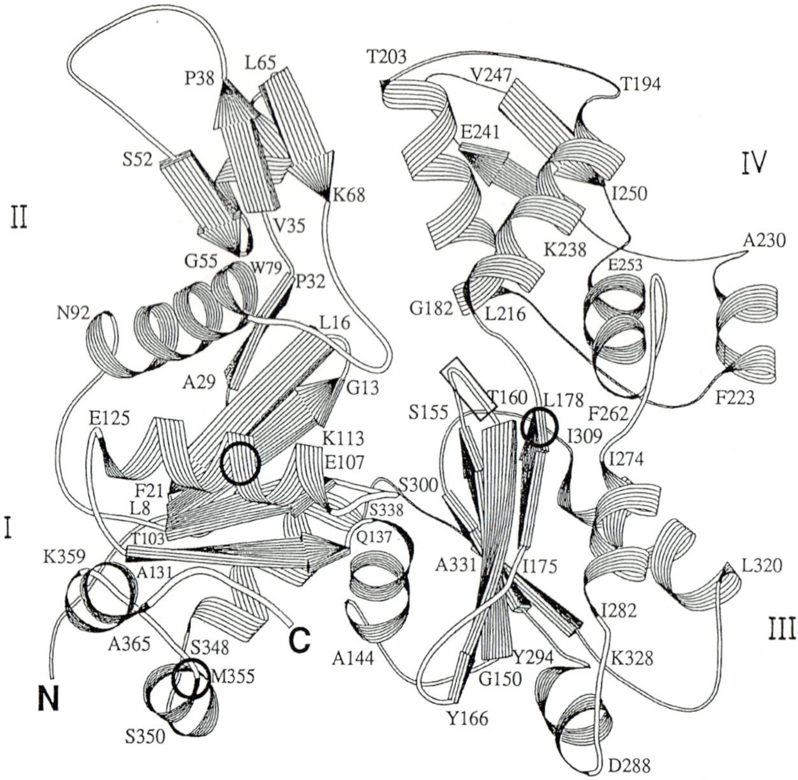

Fig. 1. Schematic representation of the three-dimensional structure of actin. Actin subdomains are indicated by I–IV. The first and last amino acid residues in the helices and sheet strands are indicated. The rectangle in subdomain III indicates residues 157–159, which interact with the γ-phosphate of ATP located in the cleft between subdomains I, II and subdomains III, IV. The *circle* in subdomain III indicates the ADP-ribose acceptor in actin (Arg-177); the *circles* in subdomain I, the putative binding sites of phalloidin. (By courtesy of Dr. W. KABSCH, Heidelberg FRG)

polymerization (50 μ*M*), inhibition of actin ATPase is observed. Second, ATP hydrolysis catalyzed by actin has been studied at actin concentrations below its critical concentration. Even at these low concentrations, which exclude actin polymerization, ADP-ribosylation decreases actin ATPase activity by more than 80%. Finally, even in the actin-DNase I complex, ADP-ribosylation impairs actin-catalyzed ATP hydrolysis (GEIPEL et al. 1990). DNase I binds G-actin with high affinity (LAZARIDES and LINDBERG 1974); therefore, in the DNase I complex, actin can be studied in a quasi-monomeric state. The mycotoxins cytochalasin B and D, which cap and sever F-actin (COOPER 1987), have been shown to stimulate G-actin ATPase about 30-fold (BRENNER and KORN 1980). GEIPEL et al. (1990) showed that ADP-ribosylation of actin inhibits the cytochalasin-induced increase in ATPase activity. Thus, in analogy with the ADP-ribosylation of G-proteins by cholera toxin and pertussis toxin, which inhibit G-protein-associated

GTP hydrolysis, the ADP-ribosylation of actin blocks actin-associated ATPase activity. According to the atomic model of actin reported by KABSCH and coworkers (1990), ATP is bound to actin in a cleft between subdomains I, II and subdomains III, IV (Fig. 1). The γ-phosphate of ATP interacts with the residues Asp-157, Gly-158, and Val-159 of actin which belong to a loop of subdomain III. It remains to be clarified whether this loop is close enough to residue Arg-177 to be influenced by the ADP-ribose moiety incorporated by the toxin.

3.3 De-ADP-Ribosylation of Actin

As shown for other mono-ADP-ribosylation reactions catalyzed, for example, by cholera toxin (CASSEL and PFEUFFER 1978) or diphtheria toxin (UCHIDA 1983), the ADP-ribosylation of actin is a reversible process. De-ADP-ribosylation of previously modified actin can be achieved in the presence of nicotinamide (10–30 m*M*) and in the absence of NAD. The reversal of ADP-ribosylation is accompanied by formation of NAD (JUST et al. 1990): Toxin-induced ADP-ribosylation and de-ADP-ribosylation of actin exhibits the identical substrate specificity, e.g., modified nonmuscle actin is de-ADP-ribosylated by C2 toxin. In contrast, α-skeletal muscle actin, which is ADP-ribosylated by *C. perfringens* iota toxin (see later), is not de-ADP-ribosylated by C2 toxin. The removal of ADP-ribose from actin is accompanied by an increase in the actin ATPase activity and reconstitutes the ability of the protein to polymerize (JUST et al. 1990).

4 Other Actin-ADP-Ribosylating Agents

Beside *C. botulinum* C2 toxin, several other clostridial actin-ADP-ribosylating toxins have been described, such as *C. perfringens* iota toxin (SIMPSON et al. 1987; STILES and WILKINS 1986a, b; SCHERING et al. 1988), *C. spiroforme* (POPOFF and BOQUET 1988; SIMPSON et al. 1989), and *C. difficile* ADP-ribosyltransferase (POPOFF et al. 1988), which is clearly distinct from *C. difficile* toxins A and B. As stated in Sect. 1, these toxins are all binary in structure and are, therefore, comparable with leukocidin (NODA et al. 1981) and *anthrax* toxin (LEPPLA 1982). Iota toxin which has been purified from the culture medium of *C. perfringens* type E (Strain NCIB 10748) is comprised of two components; M_r of 47 500 and 71 500 and isoelectric points (pI) of 5.2 and 4.2 have been determined for the enzyme component i_a and the binding component i_b, respectively (STILES and WILKINS 1986a). It has been reported that the toxicity of *C. perfringens* iota toxin is increased by proteolytic activation (ROSS et al. 1949); however, no effect of trypsin has been observed with the purified binding component, a finding which was referred to actions of endogenous proteases (STILES and WILKENS 1986b). In contrast to purified iota toxin, the binding component of *C. spiroforme* toxin has to be activitated by trypsin for full activity (POPOFF and BOQUET 1988). The enzyme component of *C. spiroforme* toxin is apparently heterogeneous, with M_r of 43 000–47 000 (POPOFF and BOQUET 1988). The ADP-ribosyltransferase produced by *C. difficile* strain (CD196) has a M_r of 43 000 and a pI of 7.8 (POPOFF et al. 1988). So far, no binding component has been detected in the *C. difficile* strain; however, the binding components of *C. spiroforme toxin* and *C. perfringens* iota toxin are able to translocate the *C. difficile* enzyme into the cell (POPOFF and BOQUET 1988). Apparently, all these toxins modify actin at the identical amino acid, namely at arginine-177 in actin. This was shown directly by protein chemical analysis in the case of iota toxin (VANDEKERCKHOVE et al. 1987) and by using the so-called back-ADP-ribosylation method in the case of the other toxins. Thereby it has been demonstrated that the prior modification of actin by C2 toxin inhibits further modification by the other enzymes (POPOFF and BOQUET 1988; SCHERING et al. 1988). However, there are clear differences between C2 toxin and the other actin-ribosylating toxins, justifying the subclassification of a group of "iota-like" actin-ADP-ribosylating toxins. For example, the toxins produced by *C. spiroforme, C. perfringens,* and *C. difficile* are immunologically related (POPOFF and BOQUET 1988; POPOFF et al. 1988). In contrast, antibodies against these toxins do not cross-react with *C. botulinum* C2 toxin. Moreover, as already mentioned, the binding components of the iota-like toxins are interchangeable, whereas this does not extend to the binding component of *C. botulinum* C2 toxin. Similarly, the enzyme component of C2 toxin is not transferred into the cell by the binding components of iota-like toxins. Apparently, the cell surface receptors for C2 toxin or iota and iota-like toxins are different because C2 toxin, but not iota-like toxins was shown to be able to enter Y-1 adrenal cells (ZEPEDA et al. 1988). Finally, there exists a striking difference in the substrate specificity between C2 toxin and iota toxin. Iota toxin is able to modify all mammalian actin isoforms, whereas C2 toxin modifies only nonmuscle actin and γ-smooth muscle actin (MAUSS et al. 1990). The same substrate specificity has been shown for the reversal of ADP-ribosylation (JUST et al. 1990). Thus, nonmuscle actin previously ADP-ribosylated by C2 toxin could be cleaved by iota toxin, whereas the iota toxin-induced ADP-ribosylation of skeletal muscle actin was not reversed by C2 toxin.

5 Toxicological Effects of Actin-ADP-Ribosylating Toxins

5.1 Toxin Effects in Animals

Whereas the single components of C2 toxin are almost nontoxic in intact animals, the combination of both components largely increases the toxicity. Most toxic is the enzyme component in combination with the trypsin-activated binding component. The LD_{50} was determined to be about 5 and 50 ng per mouse, respectively, for the intravenous and intraperitioneal route of administration (OHISHI et al. 1980a). By comparing the effects of C2 toxin with the extremely potent neurotoxin C1, SIMPSON (1982) showed that C2 toxin lacks neurotoxic activity. In rats, C2 induces hypotension, hemorrhaging in the lungs, and fluid accumulation around the lungs. Most effects of the toxin can be explained by an increase in vascular permeability. OHISHI et al. (1980b) studied the effects of C2 toxin on vascular permeability as determined by the blueing response of intradermally administered toxin after intravenous injection of Evans blue. This effects depends on the presence of both toxin components and is largely increased by prior trypsin treatment of the binding component. A maximal response (Evans blue permeability) is observed after 4–8 h with 12.5 ng of activated toxin used at a C2I:C2II ratio of 1:2 (on a microgram basis). The increase in permeability is observed even after intradermal injection of each toxin component into separate sites or after different routes of administration of the two components (OHISHI 1983a). However, the toxin effect occurs every time at the site of injection of C2II.

Recently, the effects of botulinum C2 toxin have been studied on the permeability of endothelial cell monolayers derived from porcine pulmonary arteries (SUTTORP et al. 1991). Incubation of the cell monolayer with botulinum C2 toxin resulted in a dose- and time-dependent increase in the hydraulic conductivity and decrease in the selectivity of the cell monolayer. At 100 ng C2 toxin per milliliter, the hydraulic conductivity increased tenfold. At this concentration the toxin effect occurred with a delay of about 25 min. Concomitantly, actin was ADP-ribosylated. The toxin induced the formation of interendothelial gaps, thereby possibly opening a paracellular pathway for fluid movement. The C2 toxin-induced enhancement of endothelial monolayer permeability was observed in the absence of overt cell damage (SUTTORP et al. 1991).

As another model system, the mouse intestinal loop was used. Injection of C2 toxin into the mouse intestinal loop causes fluid accumulation (OHISHI 1983b). This effect occurs after a lag period of 1–2 h, which is at least in part due to the translocation of the toxin. Fluid accumulation increases for at least 10 h. In contrast to cholera toxin, which also increases gut fluid accumulation, morphological changes which reveal the picture of an acute inflammation of the epithelium (OHISHI and ODAGIRI 1984). Severe damage to the intestinal mucosa follows, with intracellular vacuolation, desquamation and necrosis of the epithelium, and further infiltration of the lamina propria by inflammatory cells.

5.2 Cytotoxic Effects

Further studies on the toxic effects of the actin-ADP-ribosylating toxins have been done by using cell culture. The toxins induce rounding up of various types of cells. Studies with C2 toxin reveal that the cells differ in their sensitivity towards the toxin. While Vero (African green monky kidney) cells are most sensitive, with 100% rounding up at 10 ng C2 toxin per milliliter after about 24 h of treatment, for

FL (human amnion) cells about 200-fold higher concentrations are necessary to induce complete rounding up (OHISHI et al. 1984). With further incubation time (up to 48 h) most cells degenerate and are lysed. There exists a compelling amount of evidence that actin is also the substrate of the toxins in intact cells. Pretreatment of various types of cells including chicken embryo cells (REUNER et al. 1987), Vero cells (POPOFF and BOQUET 1988), Y-1 adrenal cells (ZEPEDA et al. 1988), or leukocytes (NORGAUER et al. 1988) with C2 or an iota-like toxin clearly reduces the amount of actin, which is [^{32}P]ADP-ribosylated in the cell lysate, compared with untreated cells. More direct evidence that actin is the toxin's substrate in intact cells has been obtained by using cells preloaded with [^{32}P] orthophosphoric acid (REUNER et al. 1987). Toxin treatment of these cells causes the labeling of a 42-kDa protein, which has been identified as actin by proteolytic peptide mapping. Toxin-induced rounding up of cells correlated with the ADP-ribosylation of actin in the intact cells in a time- and concentration-dependent manner.

Treatment of chicken embryo cells with C2 toxin causes destruction of the microfilament network stained by fluorescein-labeled phalloidin (REUNER et al. 1987). After treatment of the cells for only 3 h the stress fibers become condensed, shortened, and broken. Longer incubation of cells with the toxin causes a complete loss of the microfilament network. At this stage more than 95% of the cells are still vital. Whereas the microtubule system is almost unaltered by C2 toxin, the intermediate filaments are apparently also redistributed after toxin treatment. This was observed after treatment of hepatoma FAO cells with C2 toxin (WIEGERS et al. 1991). It appears, however, that the effects on the intermediate filaments are secondary and follow the changes in the microfilament network. This destruction of the microfilament network is apparently accompanied by a decrease in F-actin and increase in the G-actin content of treated cells. By using the DNase inhibition test it has been shown that the G-actin concentration increased by about threefold (AKTORIES et al. 1989). By using Triton X-100, a similar toxin-induced redistribution of G- and F-actin has been demonstrated (REUNER et al. 1987). Cytoskeleton-associated proteins, e.g., filamentous actin, are insoluble in Triton, whereas G-actin is separated in the Triton-soluble fraction. Treatment of chicken embryo cells with C2 toxin increases the Triton-soluble and decreases the Triton-insoluble actin pool. Moreover, ADP-ribosylated actin is exclusively found in the Triton-soluble fraction indicating that also in intact cells, G- but not F-actin is the primary substrate of the toxin (REUNER et al. 1987).

6 Model of the Action of Actin-ADP-Ribosylating Toxins

All these data accumulated can be summarized in a model of the cytotoxic effects of actin-ADP-ribosylating toxins (Fig. 2) (AKTORIES et al. 1989; AKTORIES and WEGNER 1989) The binary toxins bind to a receptor/acceptor at the surface of

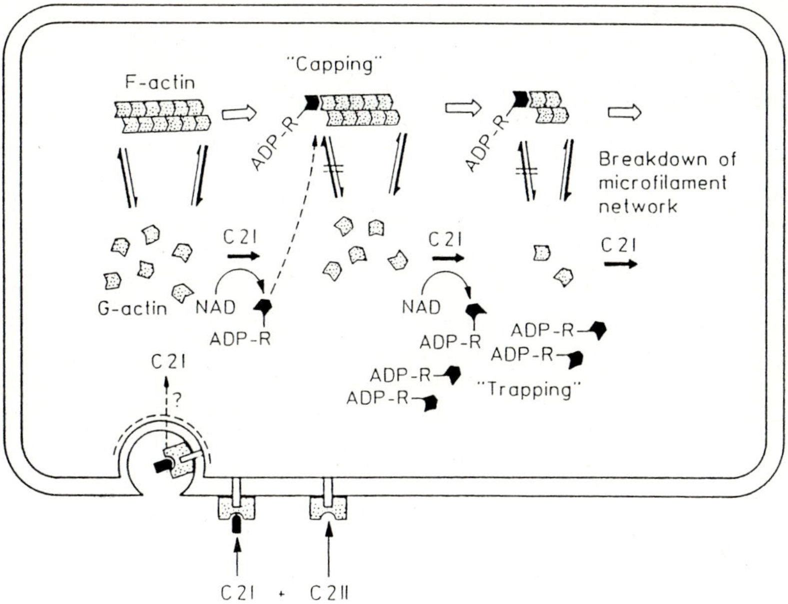

Fig. 2. Model of the action of actin-ADP-ribosylating toxins exemplified by the action of C2 toxin. The binding component C2II of the toxin attaches to an acceptor in the membrane of the target cell, thereby inducing or unmasking a binding site for the enzyme component C2I, which is transferred into the cell presumably by endocytosis. In the cell the equilibrium between polymerization and depolymerization of actin is disturbed by the toxin. ADP-ribosylation of actin inhibits its polymerizability and turns G-actin into a capping protein which binds to the fast-growing (*barbed*) ends of actin filaments. Capping of the barbed ends increases the critical concentration for actin polymerization. Since the slow-growing (*pointed*) ends of actin filaments are free, depolymerization of actin occurs at these ends. Released actin is substrate of the toxin and will be withdrawn from the treadmilling pool of actin by ADP-ribosylation. Both reactions, trapping of G-actin and capping of F-actin, will finally induce the breakdown of the microfilament network

the target cell. In the case of C2 toxin, the receptor might be a glycoprotein. Attachment of C2II demasks or induces a binding site for C2I. Most likely by receptor-mediated endocytosis, C2I is translocated into the cell where the toxin ADP-ribosylates monomeric G-actin. The modified G-actin is turned into a capping protein, which caps the fast growing end of actin filaments. At the pointed end of filaments monomeric actin is still released. The G-actin is again substrate of the toxin and is ADP-ribosylated. Since ADP-ribosylated actin has lost its ability to polymerize, it is trapped in the monomeric form and will accumulate. Both processes, inhibition of filament growth by capping and accumulation of modified G-actin by trapping, disturb the dynamic equilibrium between G- and F-actin and will finally result in the destruction of the microfilament network.

7 Actin-ADP-Ribosylating Toxins as Tools

7.1 Toxin Effects on Neutrophil Activation

For many years, the mycotoxins phalloidin and the subtypes of cytochalasin, which act by either stimulating (phalloidin) or inhibiting (cytochalasin) actin polymerization, have been used as tools to elucidate the physiological role of actin in muscle and nonmuscle cells (COOPER 1987). Recent studies have shown that also the actin-ADP-ribosylating toxins are instrumental in the physiological functions of actin. For example, the activation of neutrophils by chemotactic agents like *N*-formyl peptides, complement C5a, or leukotriene B_4 causes cellular responses such as cell shape change, adhesion, migration, degranulation, and phagocytosis. Apparently all these events depend on the restructuring of the cytoskeleton and are suggested to be associated with changes in the state of actin polymerization. In this model system it has been shown that botulinum C2 toxin inhibited the random migration and the migration stimulated by *N*-formyl peptides, complement C5a, and leukotriene B_4 (NORGAUER et al. 1988). These findings are in agreement with the view that an intact function of actin is crucial for migration of cells. The superoxide-producing membrane-bound NADPH oxidase of neutrophils, which plays an important role in microbicidal acitivity, is apparently also regulated by processes involving cytoskeleton proteins (OMANN et al. 1987). Similarly, as observed with cytochalasin B, botulinum C2 toxin treatment of neutrophils increases the *N*-formyl peptide-stimulated superoxide anion production 1.5- to 5-fold (NORGAUER et al. 1988; AL-MOHANNA et al. 1987). The effect of the toxin occurs in a time- and concentration-dependent manner and is observed only in the presence of both components of the toxin. A maximal effect occurs with 2 μg C2 toxin per milliliter (C2I:C2II = 1:4) after 45 min of incubation. After this time about 20% of the cellular actin is ADP-ribosylated, indicating that the modification of a minor actin pool has pronounced effects on the activation of neutrophils. By using the right-angle light scatter method and staining of F-actin with rhodamine-phalloidin, it has been shown that C2 toxin prevents the *N*-formyl peptide-induced increase in actin polymerization and finally completely depletes neutrophils of F-actin (NORGAUER et al. 1989). Therefore, C2 toxin was used to study the role of the actin cytoskeleton on *N*-formyl-peptide receptor dynamics in human neutrophils. It has been demonstrated that the complete loss of F-actin does not influence the association and dissociation kinetics of *N*-formyl peptides to the receptor. Furthermore, under these conditions the receptor endocytosis is slower but still possible. These findings argue against the recent hypothesis that F-actin plays a major role in *N*-formyl peptide kinetics or receptor endocytosis.

7.2 Toxin Effects on Exocytosis

Botulinum C2 toxin was used to study the role of actin in exocytosis. In neutrophils, treatment with C2 toxin increases the *N*-formyl peptide-stimulated release of *N*-acetylglucosaminidase by 100%–200% and of vitamin B_{12}-binding protein by about 150%, whereas the basal release is not affected by the toxin (NORGAUER et al. 1988). These findings reveal that actin is involved in exocytotic processes. Further studies on the role of actin in exocytosis were performed with PC-12 cells (MATTER et al. 1989). Pretreatment of PC-12 cells with botulinum C2 toxin for 4–8 h at 20 °C increases carbachol-, K^+-, and A23187-induced but not basal noradrenaline release maximally by about 1.5- to 3-fold. Concomitantly, about 75% of the cellular actin is ADP-ribosylated. This effect was interpreted to indicate that disassembly of actin filaments causes increase in the secretory response of PC-12 cells. However, toxin treatment of PC-12 cells at 37 °C affects the release of [^{3}H] norepinephrine in a biphasic manner. Whereas, short term treatment of cells for up to 1 h increases stimulated [^{3}H]norepinephrine secretion, further incubation in the presence of the toxin decreases the release stimulated by carbachol and K^+, but not by the ionophore A23187. During the stimulatory phase, 20%–50% of the cellular actin is ADP-ribosylated. When toxin treatment causes inhibition of exocytosis, more than 60% of actin is modified. Inhibition of exocytosis is also observed after treatment of mast cells with botulinum C2 toxin. BÖTTINGER et al. (1987) reported that treatment of rat mast cells with the toxin for 4 h at 37 °C inhibited the histamine release stimulated by compound 48/80 and by the mast cell degranulating peptide (MCD peptide). In contrast, histamine release stimulated by the calcium ionophore A23187 was not affected by C2 toxin.

7.3 Toxin Effects on Smooth Muscle Contraction

Recently, the effect of botulinum C2 toxin has been studied on the contraction of the guinea pig ileum plexus myentericus longitudinal muscle preparation (MAUSS et al. 1989). It has been shown that C2 toxin inhibits the muscle contraction induced by electrical stimulation in a time- and concentration-dependent manner. Again the effect occurs with a time lag (1 h) and depends on the presence of both toxin components indicating the specificity of the action of the toxin. Smooth muscle contractility is inhibited by about 60% after 4 h of incubation with 1.7 μg C2I and 6.7 μg C2II per milliliter. Under these conditions about 55% of the modifiable smooth muscle actin is ADP-ribosylated. Several findings indicate that this inhibitory effect of C2 toxin is caused by direct action on the smooth muscle cell. First, C2 toxin also inhibits the muscle contraction induced by carbachol or bradykinin. Second, the contraction of the muscle preparation is also impaired when the stimulation of the smooth muscle is caused by direct muscle membrane depolarization after suppression of acetylcholine release by normorphine. Finally, also the contraction induced by Ba^{2+} ions, which are known to affect the smooth muscle cells via a direct action, is inhibited by toxin treatment of the ileum muscle preparation. In consideration of the findings that C2 toxin ADP-ribosylates monomeric G-actin but not polymerized F-actin these data may suggest that G-actin or a G-actin/F-actin transition is involved in the regulation of smooth muscle contraction.

8 Conclusions

Studies from recent years largely increased our knowledge about the mechanisms by which various clostridial toxins which ADP-ribosylate actin elicit their cytotoxic effects on eukaryotic cells. Several interesting questions remain to be clarified : (1) The primary structures of the actin ADP-ribosylating toxins are unknown. It would be most fascinating to compare the structure/function relationship among the various ADP-ribosyltransferases. (2) The binding of the toxins to the eukaryotic cell surface and their translocation into cells is still obscure. (3) The intracellular actions of the toxins, e.g., the roles of actin-binding proteins such as gelsolin or profilin in this process have to be defined. (4) Further studies are necessary to delineate the surprising substrate specificity of C2 toxin. Finally, the impact of the actin-ADP-ribosylating toxins in the general pathogenicity of most of the clostridia producing these toxins is unclear. On the other hand, in spite of these still-open questions, it appears that the novel family of clostridial ADP-ribosylating toxins are already useful instruments with which to study the function of their target protein actin.

Acknowledgements. Studies performed in the authors' laboratory reported herein were supported by the Deutsche Forschungsgemeinschaft (Ak 6/1–1, Ak 6/1–2), Sonderforschungsbereich 249, and the Fonds der Chemischen Industrie.

Notes added in proof: Recently, the mono-ADP-ribosylation of actin by endogenous ADP-ribosyltransferases from rat brain has been described (S. MATSUYAMA and S. TSUYAMA (1991) J Neurochem 57: 1380–1387). The gelsolin-actin complexes are apparently substrates for ADP-ribosylation by *C. botulinum* C2 toxin and *C. perfringens* iota toxin (M. WILLE, I. JUST, A. WEGNER and K. AKTORIES (1992) J Biol Chem, 267: 50–55). By using *C. botulinum C2* toxin, REUNER et al. (FEBS Lett (1991) 286: 100–104) showed the autoregulatory control of the actin synthesis in cultured rat hepatocytes. Two recent publications (GRIMMINGER et al. (1991) J Biol Chem 266: 19276–19282; GRIMMINGER et al. (1991) Mol Pharmacol 40: 563–571) report on the effects of *C. botulinum* C2 toxin on the signal transduction in neutrophils.

References

Aktories K (1990) Clostridial ADP-ribosyltransferase—modification of low molecular weight GTP-binding proteins and of actin by clostridial toxins. Med Microbiol Immunol 179: 123–136

Aktories K, Wegner A (1989) ADP-ribosylation of actin by clostridial toxins. J Cell Biol 109: 1385–1387

Aktories K, Bärmann M, Ohishi I, Tsuyama S, Jakobs KH, Habermann E (1986a) Botulinum C2 toxin ADP-ribosylates actin. Nature 322: 390–392

Aktories K, Ankenbauer T, Schering B, Jakobs KH (1986b) ADP-ribosylation of platelet actin by botulinum C2 toxin. Eur J Biochem 161: 155–162

Aktories K, Weller U, Chhatwal GS (1987) *Clostridium botulinum* type C produces a novel ADP-ribosyltransferase distinct from botulinum C2 toxin. FEBS Lett 212: 109–113

Aktories K, Just I, Rosenthal W (1988) Different types of ADP-ribose protein bonds formed by botulinum C2 toxin, botulinum ADP-ribosyltransferase C3 and pertussis toxin. Biochem Biophys Res Commun 156: 361–367

Aktories K, Reuner K-H, Presek P, Bärmann M (1989) Botulinum C2 toxin treatment increases the G-actin pool in intact chicken cells: a model for the cytopathic action of actin-ADP-ribosylating toxins. Toxicon 27: 989–993

AL-Mohanna FA, Ohishi I, Hallett MB (1987) Botulinum C2 toxin potentiates activation of the neutrophil oxidase. FEBS Lett 219: 40–44

Brenner SL, Korn ED (1980) The effects of cytochalasins on actin polymerization and actin ATPase provide insights into the mechanism of polymerization. J Biol Chem 255: 841–844

Böttinger H, Reuner KH, Aktories K (1987) Inhibition of histamine release from rat mast cells by botulinum C2 toxin. Int Archs Allergy Appl Immunol 84: 380–384

Cassel D, Pfeuffer T (1978) Mechanism of cholera toxin action: covalent modification of the guanyl nucleotide-binding protein of the adenylate cyclase system. Proc Natl Acad Sci USA 75: 2669–2673

Cooper JM (1987) Effects of cytochalasin and phalloidin on actin. J Cell Biol 105: 1473–1478

Eklund MW, Poysky FT (1972) Activation of a toxic component of *Clostridium botulinum* types C and D by trypsin. Appl Microbiol 24: 108–113

Eklund MW, Poysky FT, Reed SM, Smith CA (1971) Bacteriophage and the toxigenicity of *Clostridium botulinum* type C. Science 172: 480–482

Eklund MW, Poysky FT, Reed SM (1972) Bacteriophage and the toxigenicity of *Clostridium botulinum* type D. Nature [New Biol] 235: 16–17

Geipel U, Just I, Schering B, Haas D, Aktories K (1989) ADP-ribosylation of actin causes increase in the rate of ATP exchange and inhibition of ATP hydrolysis. Eur J Biochem 179: 229–232

Geipel U, Just I, Aktories K (1990) Inhibition of cytochalasin D-stimulated G-actin ATPase by ADP-ribosylation with *Clostridium perfringens* iota toxin. Biochem J 266: 335–339

Gill DM (1977) Mechanism of action of cholera toxin. Adv Cyclic Nucleotide Res 8: 85–118

Holmes KC, Popp D, Gebhard W, Kabsch W (1990) Atomic model of the actin filament. Nature 347: 44–49

Hsia JA, Tsai S-C, Adamik R, Yost DA, Hewlett EL, Moss J (1985) Amino acid-specific ADP-ribosylation. J Biol Chem 260: 16187–16191

Just I, Geipel U, Wegner A, Aktories K (1990) De-ADP-ribosylation of actin by *Clostridium perfringens* iota-toxin and *Clostridium botulinum* C2 toxin. Eur J Biochem 192: 723–727

Kabsch W, Mannherz HG, Suck D, Pai EF, Holmes KC (1990) Atomic structure of the actin:DNase I complex. Nature 347: 37–44

Lazarides E, Lindberg U (1974) Actin is the naturally occurring inhibitor of deoxyribonuclease I. Proc Nat Acad Sci 71: 4742–4746

Leppla SH (1982) Anthrax toxin edema factor: bacterial adenylate cyclase that increases cyclic AMP concentrations in eukaryotic cells. Proc Natl Acad Sci USA 79: 3162–3166

Matter K, Dreyer F, Aktories K (1989) Actin involvement in exocytosis from PC12 cells: studies on the influence of botulinum C2 toxin on stimulated noradrenaline release. J Neurochem 52: 370–376

Mauss S, Koch G, Kreye VAW, Aktories K (1989) Inhibition of the contraction of the isolated longitudinal muscle of the guinea-pig ileum by botulinum C2 toxin: evidence for a role of G/F-actin transition in smooth muscle contraction. Naunyn Schmiedebergs Arch Pharmacol 340: 345–351

Mauss S, Chaponnier C, Just I, Aktories K, Gabbiani G (1990) ADP-ribosylation of actin isoforms by *C. botulinum* C2 toxin and *C. perfringens* iota toxin. Eur J Biochem 194: 237–241

Moss J, Vaughan M (eds) (1990) ADP-ribosylating toxins and G proteins. Insight into signal transduction. American Society for Microbiology, Washington

Nakamura S, Serikawa T, Noshida S, Kozaki S, Sakaguchi G (1978) Sporulation and C_2 toxin production by *Clostridium botulinum* type C strains producing no C_1 toxin. Microbiol Immunol 22: 591–596

Noda M, Kato I, Matsuda F, Hirayama T (1981) Mode of action of staphylococcal leukocidin: relationship between binding of ^{125}I-labeled S and F components of leukocidin to rabbit polymorphnuclear leukocytes and leukocidin activity. Infect Immun 34: 362–367

Norgauer J, Kownatzki E, Seifert R, Aktories K (1988) Botulinum C2 toxin ADP-ribosylates actin and enhances O_2^- production and secretion but inhibits migration of activated human neutrophils. J Clin Invest 82: 1376–1382

Norgauer J, Just I, Aktories K, Sklar LA (1989) Influence of botulinum C2 toxin on F-actin and *N*-formyl peptide receptor dynamics in human neutrophils. J Cell Biol 109: 1133–1140

Ohishi I (1983a) Response of mouse intestinal loop to botulinum C2 toxin: enterotoxic activity induced by cooperation of nonlinked protein components. Infect Immun 40: 691–695

Ohishi I (1983b) Lethal and vascular permeability activities of botulinum C2 toxin induced by separate injection of the two toxin components. Infect Immun 40: 336–339

Ohishi I (1986) NAD-glycohydrolase activity of botulinum C2 toxin: a possible role of component I in the mode of action of the toxin. J Biochem (Tokyo) 100: 407–413

Ohishi I (1987) Activation of botulinum C2 toxin by trypsin. Infect Immun 55: 1461–1465

Ohishi I, Miyake M (1985) Binding of the two components of C2 toxin to epithelial cells and brush borders of mouse intestine. Infect Immun 48: 769–775

Ohishi I,.Odagiri Y (1984) Histopathological effect of botulinum C2 toxin on mouse intestines. Infect Immun 43: 54–58

Ohishi I, Okada Y (1986) Heterogeneities of two components of C2 toxin produced by *Clostridium botulinum* types C and D. J Gen Microbiol 132: 125–131

Ohishi I, Iwasaki M, Sakaguchi G (1980a) Purification and characterization of two components of botulinum C2 toxin. Infect Immun 30: 668–673

Ohishi I, Iwasaki M, Sakaguchi G (1980b) Vascular permeability activity of botulinum C2 toxin elicited by cooperation of two dissimilar protein components. Infect Immun 31: 890–895

Ohishi I, Miyake M, Ogura K, Nakamura S (1984) Cytopathic effect of botulinum C2 toxin on tissue-culture cell lines. FEMS Lett Microbiol 23: 281–284

Omann GM, Allen RA, Bokoch GM, Painter RG, Traynor AE, Sklar LA (1987) Signal transduction and cytoskeletal activation in the neutrophil. Physiol Rev 67: 285–322

Pollard T, Cooper JA (1986) Actin and actin-binding proteins. A critical evaluation of mechanism and functions. Annu Rev Biochem 55: 987–1035

Popoff MR, Boquet P (1988) *Clostridium spiroforme* toxin is a binary toxin which ADP-ribosylates cellular actin. Biochem Biophys Res Commun 152: 1361–1368

Popoff MR, Rubin EJ, Gill DM, Boquet P (1988) Actin-specific ADP-ribosyltransferase produced by a *Clostridium difficile* strain. Infect Immun 56: 2299–2306

Popoff MR, Boquet P, Gill DM, Eklund MW (1990) DNA sequence of exoenzyme C3, an ADP-ribosyltransferase encoded by Clostridum botulinum C and D phages. Nucl Acids Res 18: 1291

Reuner KH, Presek P, Boschek CB, Aktories K (1987) Botulinum C2 toxin ADP-ribosylates actin and disorganizes the microfilament network in intact cells. Eur J Cell Biol 43: 134–140

Ross HE, Warren ME, Barnes J (1949) *Clostridium welchii* iota toxin: its activation by trypsin. J Gen Microbiol 3: 148–152

Rubin EJ, Gill DM, Boquet P, Popoff MR (1988) Functional modification of a 21-kilodalton G protein when ADP-ribosylated by exoenzyme C3 of *Clostridium botulinum.* Mol Cell Biol 8: 418–426

Schering B, Bärmann M, Chhatwal GS, Geipel U, Aktories K (1988) ADP-ribosylation of skeletal muscle and non-muscle actin by *Clostridium perfringens* iota toxin. Eur J Biochem 171: 225–229

Simpson LL (1982) A comparison of the pharmacological properties of *Clostridium botulinum* type C1 and C2 toxins. J Pharmacol Exp Ther 223: 695–701

Simpson LL (1984) Molecular basis for the pharmacological actions of *Clostridium botulinum* type C2 toxin. J Pharmacol Exp Ther 230: 665–669

Simpson LL (1989) The binary toxin produced by *Clostridium botulinum* enters cells by receptor-mediated endocytosis to exert its pharmacologic effects. J Pharmacol Exp Ther 251: 1223–1228

Simpson LL, Stiles BG, Zapeda HH, Wilkins TD (1987) Molecular basis for the pathological actions of *Clostridium perfringens* iota toxin. Infect Immun 55: 118–122

Simpson LL, Zepeda H, Ohishi I (1988) Partial characterization of the enzymatic activity associated with the binary toxin (type C2) produced by *Clostridium botulinum.* Infect Immun 56: 24–27

Simpson LL, Stiles BG, Zepeda H, Wilkins TD (1989) Production by *Clostridium spiroforme* of an iota-like toxin that possesses mono (ADP-ribosyl) transferase activity: identification of a novel class of ADP-ribosyltransferases. Infect Immun 57: 255–261

Stiles BG, Wilkins TD (1986a) Purification and characterization of *Clostridium perfringens* iota toxin: dependence on two nonlinked proteins for biological activity. Infect Immun 54: 683–688

Stiles BG, Wilkins TD (1986b) *Clostridium perfringens* iota toxin: synergism between two proteins. Toxicon 24: 767–773

Sugii S, Kozaki S (1990) Hemagglutinating and binding properties of botulinum C2 toxin. Biochim Biophys Acta 1034: 176–179

Suttorp N, Polley M, Seybold J, Schnittler H, Aktories K (1991) ADP-ribosylation of G-actin botulinum C2 toxin increases endothelial permeability in vitro. J Chin Invest 87: 1575–1584

Tamura M, Nogimuri K, Murai S, Yajima M, Ito K, Katada T, Ui M, Ishii S (1982) Subunit structure of islet-activating protein, pertussis toxin, in conformity with the A–B model. Biochemistry 21: 5516–5522

Uchida T (1983) Diphtheria toxin. Pharmacol Ther 19: 107–122

Vandekerckhove J, Weber K (1979) The complete amino acid sequence of actins from bovine aorta, bovine heart, bovine fast skeletal muscle and rabbit slow skeletal muscle. Differentiation 14: 123–133

Vandekerckhove J, Schering B, Bärmann M, Aktories K (1987) *Clostridium perfringens* iota toxin ADP-ribosylates skeletal muscle actin in Arg-177. FEBS Lett 225: 48–52

Vandekerckhove J, Schering B, Bärmann M, Aktories K (1988) Botulinum C2 toxin ADP-ribosylates cytoplasmic β/γ-actin in arginine 177. J Biol Chem 263: 696–700

Wegner A, Aktories K (1988) ADP-ribosylated actin caps the barbed ends of actin filaments. J Biol Chem 263: 13739–13742

Weigt C, Just I, Wegner A, Aktories K (1989) Nonmuscle actin ADP-ribosylated by botulinum C2 toxin caps actin filaments. FEBS Lett 246: 181–184

Wiegers W, Just I, Müller H, Traub P, Aktories K (1991) Alteration of the cytoskeleton of mammalian cells cultured in vitro by *Clostridium botulinum* C2 toxin and C3 ADP-ribosyltransferase. Eur J Cell Biol 54: 237–245

Zepeda H, Considine RV, Smith HL, Sherwin JA, Ohishi I, Simpson LL (1988) Actions of the *Clostridium botulinum* binary toxin on the structure and function of Y-1 adrenal cells. J Pharmacol Exp Ther 246: 1183–1189

Clostridium botulinum C3 ADP-Ribosyltransferase

K. AKTORIES, C. MOHR, and G. KOCH

1 Introduction

During the last few years various clostridial ADP-ribosylating exoenzymes have been described. These exoenzymes can be divided into two groups. One group is represented by clostridial cytotoxins which are characterized by their ability to ADP-ribosylate actin. Furthermore, all these toxins are binary in structure and consist of a binding component and an unlinked ADP-ribosyltransferase. Members of this family of clostridial ADP-ribosylating toxins are *Clostridium botulinum* C2 toxin, *Clostridium perfringens* toxin, and *Clostridium spiroforme* toxin. These toxins are described in detail by AKTORIES et al., in this volume. The other group of clostridial ADP-ribosylating exoenzymes is represented by

Institut für Pharmakologie und Toxikologie der Universität des Saarlandes, 6650 Homburg, FRG

Current Topics in Microbiology and Immunology, Vol. 175

C. botulinum ADP-ribosyltransferase C3 and by the novel ADP-ribosylating *Clostridium limosum* exoenzyme.

C. botulinum ADP-ribosyltransferase C3 was discovered in our laboratory by serendipity. In order to find high-producer strains for *C. botulinum* C2 toxin, we screened several strains of *C. botulinum* type C and D. By testing the ADP-ribosyltransferase activities of culture supernatants in the presence of human platelet membranes and [^{32}P]NAD, we observed that the culture filtrates of certain strains not only caused the ADP-ribosylation of the 42-kDa actin catalyzed by C2 toxin but also induced the labeling of 20- to 24-kDa proteins. The novel exoenzyme responsible for this ADP-ribosylation reaction was called C3 in order to distinguish it from *C. botulinum* neurotoxins and from C2 toxins (Aktories et al. 1987). As C3 is produced by *C. botulinum* strains which also synthesize botulinum neurotoxins in parallel, a lot of confusion about the relationship of these clostridial agents arose. Some investigators ascribed the ADP-ribosyltransferase activity of C3 to the action of neurotoxins. It is now generally accepted that C3 is neither structurally, immunologically, nor functionally related to the neurotoxins. Whereas the "mystery" of the biochemical basis of the action of botulinum neurotoxins remains unsolved, our knowledge about the exoenzyme C3, its eukaryotic substrates, and the functional consequences of the ADP-ribosylation has been largely increased during the last few years. The review of these data is the main topic of this chapter.

2 Origin and Purification of *C. botulinum* C3 ADP-Ribosyltransferase

C3 ADP-ribosyltransferase is produced by many strains of *C. botulinum* types C and D (Aktories et al. 1987, 1988a; Rubin et al. 1988). Whereas the structural gene of *C. botulinum* C2 toxin is most likely chromosomally encoded, C3 and the neurotoxins C1 and D are phage-encoded (Eklund and Poysky 1972;

```
1
AYSNTYQEFTNIDQAKAWGNAQYKKYGLSKSEKEAIVSYT
41
KSASEINGKLRQNKGVINGFPSNLJKQVELLDKSFNKMKT
81
PENIMLFRGDDPAYLGTEFQNTLLNSNGTINKTAFEKAKA
121
KFLNKDRLEYGYISTSLMNVSQFAGRPIITKFKVAKGSKA
161
GYIDPISAFAGQLEMLLDRHSTYHIDDMRLSSDGKQIIIT
201
ATMMGTAINPK
```

Fig. 1. Amino acid sequence deduced from the cDNA of *C. botulinum* ADP-ribosyltransferase C3. (From Popoff et al. 1990)

EKLUND et al. 1972; RUBIN et al. 1988). Recently, POPOFF and coworkers (1990) reported the sequences of the DNA of C and D phages encoding C3. According to this report C3 is comprised of 211 amino acids with M_r of 23546 (Fig. 1). The coding sequence of type C and D phages are identical with the exception of two nucleotide exchanges in the untranslated region. From these studies the existence of a precursor protein has been proposed; however, its amino acid sequence is still unknown.

C3 was purified from the supernatant of 48-h cultures of *C. botulinum* type C (AKTORIES et al. 1988a). After ammonium sulfate (70%) precipitation, the dissolved protein was desalted by gel filtration with Sephadex G25 and then applied onto DEAE-Sephadex A 50 chromatography. The flow through contains about 90% pure C3. For further purification to apparent homogeneity, the C3 preparation was simply heated for 2 min at 90 °C, and precipitating contaminants were separated by centrifugation. As the heat treatment reduces the yield, we now purify C3 by using gel filtration of Sephacryl S 100 as the last step.

3 The Relationship of *C. botulinum* C3 ADP-Ribosyltransferase to Botulinum Neurotoxins

Different groups have shown that preparations of botulinum neurotoxins C1 and D contain ADP-ribosyltransferase activity modifying low-mass GTP-binding proteins (OHASHI and NARUMIYA 1987; MATSUOKA et al. 1989; KIKUCHI et al. 1988). Particularly high ADP-ribosyltransferase activity has been observed with commercially available neurotoxins which were rather crude preparations. Several findings indicate that C3 is a contaminant of those toxin preparations. C3 possesses a specific ADP-ribosyltransferase activity about 1000 times higher than that of the neurotoxin preparations (AKTORIES and FREVERT 1987). Apparently, C3 ADP-ribosyltransferase is not only different from but even unrelated to botulinum neurotoxins. Thus, C3 differs not only in molecular mass from botulinum neurotoxins (M_r 150000; HABERMANN and DREYER 1986) but also in that antibodies produced against C3 which block the C3-induced ADP-ribosylation do not cross-react with neurotoxins (RÖSENER et al. 1987). These antibodies block the neurotoxin-induced ADP-ribosylation of low-mass GTP-binding proteins but not the toxin-induced inhibition of neurotransmitter release from chromaffin cells (ADAM-VIZI et al. 1988). On the other hand, anti-neurotoxin D antibody, which blocks the neurotoxicity, shows no effect on the ADP-ribosyltransferase activity elicited by unpurified neurotoxin D (ADAM-VIZI et al. 1988). Final evidence for the misrelation of C3 and neurotoxins can be derived from the recent reports on the DNA sequence of C3 also showing that the localization of the structural gene of C3 is clearly distinct from the locus of the neurotoxin gene (POPOFF et al. 1990). Recently, MORIISHI et al. (1990) confirmed our findings that neurotoxin D does not possess ADP-ribosyltransferase activity by separating the toxin from the ADP-ribosyltransferase, using hydroxyapatite and immunoaffinity chromatography.

4 Characterization of *C. botulinum* C3 ADP-Ribosyltransferase

C3 has a molecular weight of about 25000 on SDS-PAGE and is a very basic protein with a IP of about 10 (JUST, unpublished observation), a property allowing simple purification by anion exchange chromatography. Several findings indicate that C3 catalyzes a mono-ADP-ribosylation reaction: (1) The labeling of eukaryotic proteins induced by C3 in the presence of [^{32}P]NAD is decreased by addition of unlabeled NAD but not by ADP-ribose (AKTORIES et al. 1987, 1988a). (2) ADP-ribosylation increases the molecular weights of modified proteins by about 1000, indicating that one, but not more, ADP-ribose moieties are incorporated (AKTORIES et al. 1987). (3) *Crotalus adamanteus* phosphodiesterase is able to cleave the incorporated ADP-ribose, releasing AMP (AKTORIES et al. 1988a). As known for other bacterial ADP-ribosyltransferases, C3 possesses NAD glycohydrolase activity, thereby cleaving NAD into ADP-ribose and nicotinamide (AKTORIES et al. 1988a). The K_m of the C3-induced ADP-ribosylation for NAD is about 1 μM, and the pH optimum for the reaction was found to be about 7.5. As observed with other ADP-ribosylating toxins such as cholera toxin or C2 toxin, the ADP-ribosylation induced by C3 is a reversible reaction (HABERMANN et al. 1991). In the absence of NAD, at low pH and in the presence of nicotinamide, C3 de-ADP-ribosylates previously modified Rho protein, thereby forming NAD. The pH optimum for the reverse reaction of ADP-ribosylation is pH 5.5.

5 GTP-Binding Proteins, Substrates of C3 ADP-Ribosyltransferase

For unknown reasons, all bacterial ADP-ribosylating toxins so far studied modify nucleotide-binding proteins. For example, cholera (CASSEL and PFEUFFER 1978) and pertussis toxins (BOKOCH et al. 1983; UI 1990) modify G-proteins involved in signal transduction. Diphtheria toxin (HONJO et al. 1968; COLLIER 1990) and *Pseudomonas aeruginosa* exotoxin A (IGLEWSKI and KABAT 1975; WICK and IGLEWSKI 1990) ADP-ribosylate elongation factor 2, which is also a GTP-binding protein. *C. botulinum* C2 toxin, *C. perfringens* iota toxin, and *C. spiroforme* toxin belong to the family of actin-ADP-ribosylating toxins (AKTORIES et al. 1986a, b; SCHERING et al. 1988; POPOFF and BOQUET 1988). Actin is not a GTP-binding protein but binds ATP.

Recently, it has been shown that C3 ADP-ribosylates the Rho and Rac proteins. These protein substrates belong to the family of "small" GTP-binding proteins having molecular masses of about 20–26 kDa. The best-studied examples of these GTP-binding proteins are those which are encoded by the *ras* genes (H-, N-, and K-*ras*; BARBACID 1987). These genes respective proteins have been the focus of intensive research because mutant alleles of the genes are frequently found in human and rodent tumors. The small GTP-binding proteins are encoded by a superfamily of related genes. So far at least 30 GTP-binding proteins have been described. Among these are Rap (1A, B, and 2; PIZON et al. 1988), Rab (1–6; TOUCHOT et al. 1987), Ral (A and B; CHARDIN and TAVITIAN 1986); Rho (A, B, and C; MADAULE and AXEL 1985), Rac (1 and 2; DIDSBURY et al. 1989), and others. Recently, the crystal structure of the H-Ras protein has been reported (PAI et al. 1989; DE VOS et al. 1988), suggesting that probably all GTP-binding proteins, including elongation factors and signal-transducing G-proteins, share a common structural design (Fig. 2). A common feature of these proteins is their regulation by a GTPase cycle (BOURNE et al. 1991). Similar to G-proteins (PFEUFFER and HELMREICH 1988), the small GTP-binding proteins are inactive in the GDP-bound form and are activated by a GDP/GTP exchange (HALL 1990). Then, the GTP-bound species is suggested to interact with the respective effector. The activated state of the regulatory protein is terminated by hydrolysis of the bound GTP by an inherent GTPase activity. Recently it has been shown that the associated GTPase activity is very low but can be stimulated by a GTPase-activating protein (GAP) by more than 100-fold (TRAHEY and MCCORMICK 1987). Apparently, these GAPs are specific for the individual GTP-binding proteins. Thus, the *ras* GAP has a molecular weight of about 130 kDa, whereas the *rho* GAP exhibits a molecular mass of about 29 kDa (GARRETT et al. 1989). Furthermore, additional proteins have been identified which are apparently involved

```
1                         26                        51
MTEY--KLVVVGAGGVGKSALTIQLIQ NHFVDEYDPTIEDSYRKQVVIDGET CLLDILDTAGQEEY
*AAIRK***I**D*AC**TC*L*VFSK DQ*PEV*V**VFEN*VADIEV**KQ VE*ALW******D*

            76                        101
SAMRDQYMRTG EGFLCVFAINNTKSFEDIHQYREQI KRVKDSDDVPMVLVGNKCDL
DRL*PLSYPDT DVI*MC*S*DSPD***N*PEKWTPE VK-HFCPN**II*****KD*RNDE-HTRRE

          126                       151
   AA-RTV ESRQAQDLARSY-GIPYIETSAKTRQ GVEDAFYTLVREIRQHKLRKLNPPD
LAKMKQEPV KPEEGRNM*NAIGAFG*M*C****KD **REV*EMAT*AAL*ARRG*KKSG

176
ESGPGCMSCKCVLS
        *LVL
```

Fig. 2. Alignment of H-Ras protein sequence with RhoA. In p21^{ras} conserved regions involved in guanine nucleotide binding are residues 10–17, 53–62, 112–119, and 144–146. The so-called effector region is comprised of residues 32–40 (PAI et al. 1989; BOURNE et al. 1991). The C-terminal cysteine is posttranslationally modified by polyisoprenylation (for details see text)

in the regulation of the GTP-binding proteins. UEDA et al. (1990) discovered a protein with M_r 27 000 on SDS-PAGE in bovine brain cytosol that inhibits the dissociation of GDP from the Rho (A and B) proteins but is inactive for other GTP-binding proteins such as H-Ras. On the other hand, two GDP dissociation stimulators have been described by the same group (ISOMURA et al. 1990). These proteins specifically increase the GDP-GTP exchange rate and are specific for Rho proteins. A similar nucleotide exchange factor and GDP-releasing protein, which are specific for Ras proteins, have been detected recently (DOWNWARD et al. 1990; WOLFMAN and MACARA 1990). Thus, it appears that the active state of some low-molecular mass GTP-binding proteins is controlled by several different regulatory proteins in a complex manner.

6 *Rho* and *Rac* Proteins

It appears that *rho* genes are present in all eukaryotic cells. The *rho* gene was first detected in *Aplysia* (MADAULE and AXEL 1985). At least three *rho* genes (*rho*A, B, C) have been recognized in human tissues that are about 85% homologous to each other (MADAULE and AXEL 1985). The homology in respect to *Aplysia rho* and H-*ras* is about 85% and 35% respectively. Whereas *rho* A and *rho* C encode proteins with 193 amino acids, the *rho* B protein consists of 196 amino acids (CHARDIN et al. 1988; YERAMIAN et al. 1987; Fig. 3). Since mutant Ras proteins appear to be involved in cell transformation, studies have been carried out to discover whether this is also true for Rho proteins. For this purpose variants of Rho A have been used which have glycine and leucine

```
1                              31                             61
MAAIRKKLVIVGDGACGKTCLLIVFSKDQF PEVYVPTVFENYVADIEVDGKQVELALWDT AGQEDY
*********V*****************E*  ****************************** ******
****************************** ************I***************** ******
*Q**--*C*V****AV*******SYTTNA* *GE*I****D**S*NVMV***P*N*G**** ******
*Q**--*C*V****AV*******SYTTNA* *GE*I****D**S*NVMV*S*P******** ******

                         91                             121
DRLRPLSYPDTDVILMCFSIDSPD SLENIPEKWTPEVKHFCPNVPIILVGNKKD LRNDEHTRRE
*******************V**** *********V***************A**** **S***V*T*
************************ ****************************** **Q*******
*********Q***F*I***LV**A *F**VRA**Y***R*H***T******T*L* **D*KD*IEK
*********Q***F*I***LV**A *Y**VRA**F***R*H**ST******T*L* **D*KD*IEK

                     151                            181
LAKMKQEPVKPEEGRDMANR IGAFGYMECSAKTKDGVREVFEMATRAALQ ARRGKKKSG---CLVL
**R******RTDD**A**V* *Q*YD*L*******E*******T******* K*Y*SQNGCINC*K**
*********RS********* *S****L*******E************G** V*KN*RRR*---*PI*
*KEK*LT*ITYPQ*LA**KE ***VK*L****L*QR*LKT**DEAIRAV*C PPPVKKR*RK--**L*
*KEK*LA*ITYPQ*LAL*KE *DSVK*L****L*QR*LKT**DEAIRAV*C PQPTRQQ*RA--*S**
```

Fig. 3. Alignment of amino acid sequences of RhoA with those of RhoB, RhoC (YERAMIAN et al. 1987; CHARDIN et al. 1988), Rac 1, and Rac 2 (DIDSBURY et al. 1989)

instead of glutamine in positions 14 and 64, respectively (AVRAHAM and WEINBERG 1989). These *rho* mutations mirror the replacements responsible for oncogenic activation of the related *ras*-encoded p21 proteins. Whereas those *rho* mutants showed no transformation activity, overexpression of normal *rho* A in rat-1 and 3T3 fibroblasts resulted in colonies showing altered growth regulation. Injections of these transfected cells into athymic nude mice resulted in the formation of tumors (AVRAHAM 1990).

In yeast (*Saccharomyces cerevisiae*) two *RHO* (*RHO1* and *RHO2*) genes have been detected which are 53% identical (MADAULE et al. 1987). *RHO1* gene is 70% homologous to *Aplysia rho*. Whereas *RHO1* is necessary for cell viability, *RHO2* is not an essential gene. Mutation of Glu-68 in *RHO1* to His blocks sporulation of yeast. All Rho proteins identified so far are substrates of C3 (AKTORIES et al. 1989; KICHUCHI et al. 1988; BRAUN et al. 1989; NARUMIYA et al. 1988; CHARDIN et al. 1989; HOSHIJIMA et al. 1990).

Recently the Rac 1 and 2 proteins have been recognized as substrates of C3 (DIDSBURY et al. 1989). The *rac* genes are about 90% identical and share about 30% homology with *ras*. The homology of *rac* with *rho* is somewhat higher with about 60%. Rac 1 and Rac 2 consist of 192 amino acids with molecular masses of 21 450 and 21 429 Da, respectively (DIDSBURY et al. 1989). Whereas *rac1* is apparently localized in several different tissues, the *rac2* transcript was only detected in myeloid cells (HL-60, U 937, leukocytes). In human platelet membranes the Rac 1 protein has been detected (POLAKIS et al. 1989).

Several small GTP-binding proteins share the motif CAAX (C, cysteine; A, aliphatic amino acid; X, any amino acid) at the C-terminus (Fig. 2 and Fig. 3). Recently it has been shown that this motif at the C-terminus is required for posttranslational polyisoprenylation of Ras proteins (HANCOCK et al. 1989). The cysteine at position 4 from the C-terminus is farnesylated, and concomitantly the three AAX amino acids are cleaved with subsequent carboxymethylation of the cysteine. Moreover, further palmitoylation occurring at cysteine located upstream from the CAAX motif is apparently a prerequisite for the interaction of Ha- and N-Ras with the membrane. Since the Rac proteins also possess the CAAX motif at the C-terminal end, studies have been carried out to ascertain whether Rac 1 and Rac 2 are also posttranslationally modified by polyisoprenylation. Therefore, COS cells were transfected with *rac* 1 and *rac* 2 cDNA and the expressed proteins were subsequently labeled with [^{3}H]mevalonic acid. Using this assay, isoprenylation was observed in *rac* protein associated with the particulate cell fractions (DIDSBURY et al. 1990). Furthermore, evidence has been presented that also *Rho* proteins are modified by polyisoprenylation. These studies were performed with *Xenopus laevis* oocytes (MOHR et al. 1990). After microinjection of recombinant *rho*A protein into the oocytes, the GTP-binding proteins undergo an intracellular translocation process. Within about 1 h, Rho is dislocated into the particular fraction of oocytes. This process is blocked by the hydroxymethylglutaryl-CoA inhibitor lovastatin (mevinolin), which inhibits the formation of mevalonic acid and subsequent formation of isoprene residues. Furthermore, preliminary studies have shown that recombinant RhoA and -B, and also the respective ADP-ribosylated proteins, are specifically labeled in the presence of *X. laevis* oocyte lysate and [^{14}C]isopentenylpyrophosphate (MOHR and AKTORIES, unpublished observation). Thus, the Rho and Rac proteins appear to undergo posttranslational modification similar to that reported for Ras proteins.

Since Rho/Rac proteins appear to be ubiquitous proteins, C3 ADP-ribosylates 21- to 24-kDa proteins in all cells and tissues studied so far. Studies were performed in human platelets (AKTORIES et al. 1988a) and neutrophils (BOKOCH et al. 1988; MEGE et al. 1988), murine brain, kidney, spleen, heart, testis, and lung (MORII et al. 1988; RUBIN et al. 1988; MATSUOKA et al. 1989), porcine brain (BRAUN et al. 1989), and bovine brain (KIKUCHI et al. 1988). Whereas high concentrations of the C3 substrates were detected in rat brain (40 pmol/mg), adrenal gland (24 pmol/mg), kidney (21 pmol/mg), and thymus (20 pmol/mg), relatively low concentrations of the substrates were found in heart tissue (MORII et al. 1988). C3-catalyzed ADP-ribosylation of 21- to 24-kDa proteins has been observed in various cell lines including 1321 N1 astrocytoma cells (QUILLIAM et al. 1988), neuroblastoma glioma hybrid cells (AKTORIES et al. 1987), N18, N1E115, NS20Y, C6 (MATSUOKA et al. 1989), GH3 (BANGA et al. 1988), HL-60 (BANGA et al. 1988; DIDSBURY et al. 1989), S49 lymphoma cells (AKTORIES et al. 1987), NIH 3T3, NRK, CV-1, HEp-2, HeLa (RUBIN et al. 1988), and PC12 cells (MATSUOKA et al. 1987, 1989; RUBIN et al. 1988; NISHIKI et al. 1990). Furthermore, C3 ADP-ribosylated proteins of about 21 kDa in *X. laevis* oocytes (RUBIN et al. 1988) and *Drosophila melanogaster* (QUILLIAM et al. 1988). In most tissues at least two proteins of about 21 and 24 kDa are labeled by C3, and sometimes a third labeled protein of about 26 kDa is seen after extended autoradiography. The precise nature of the C3 substrates in the various tissues and cell lines has not been determined, and many of these studies were performed with the C3 exoenzyme found as a contaminant in botulinum neurotoxin type C and D preparations.

The cellular localization of the C3 target proteins is different in various types of cells and tissues. Whereas in neutrophils and erythrocytes the C3 substrate is mainly associated with the membrane (BOKOCH et al. 1988), in NRK cells more than 80% of the label is found in the cytosolic fraction (unpublished observation). In bovine adrenal gland the C3 substrate is found almost equally distributed between membrane and cytosolic fractions (NARUMIYA et al. 1988). TOKI et al. (1989) studied the localization of the C3 substrates in rat liver cells. Most of the C3 substrate was found in the Golgi fraction, with a smaller amount in the rough endoplasmic reticulum. Moreover, further analysis of the Golgi fraction revealed that most of the C3 substrate was detected in a fraction representing secretory vesicles.

7 Regulation of C3-Induced ADP-Ribosylation by Guanine Nucleotides

The ADP-ribosylation of eukaryotic proteins by C3 is regulated by guanine nucleotides and divalent cations. Without free Mg^{2+} poor ADP-ribosylation of Rho/Rac proteins is detectable. At low concentrations of Mg^{2+} (100–500 μ*M*) the ADP-ribosylation is maximal, whereas high concentrations (1 m*M*) of the divalent cations decrease the C3-catalyzed ADP-ribosylation. In the absence of divalent cations, guanine nucleotides (GTP, GTPγS, and GDP) increase the ADP-ribosylation (Aktories et al. 1988a; Habermann et al. 1991). Without Mg^{2+} the GTP-binding proteins probably lose their nucleotides and denature. Thus the addition of guanine nucleotides stabilizes the C3 substrates and increases the ADP-ribosylation. The stabilizing effects of guanine nucleotides are most likely responsible for the findings that the addition of GTP, GTPγS, and GDP, but not GMP or ATP, prevent the deactivation of the C3 substrates of human platelet membranes by heat treatment (10 min, 55 °C) (Aktories et al. 1988). Similarly, guanine nucleotides prevented the N-ethylmaleimide-induced deactivation (Rubin et al. 1988).

Beside the stabilizing effect, guanine nucleotides appear to regulate the ADP-ribosylation in a different manner. It appears that the GDP-bound form is the primary substrate of the C3-induced ADP-ribosylation of Rho protein. Purified Rho protein is usually GDP bound. When GDP is exchanged against GTP or GTPγS by treating the Rho/Rac proteins with EDTA in the presence of the nucleotides, the rate of the ADP-ribosylation is largely decreased compared with GDP. The de-ADP-ribosylation of modified Rho protein is similarly regulated by guanine nucleotides. The rate of de-ADP-ribosylation catalyzed by C3 is largely increased, with the modified C3 substrate having GDP-bound (Habermann et al. 1991). In contrast, Williamson et al. (1990) reported that RhoA protein purified from bovine brain was most effectively ADP-ribosylated in the presence of GTP of GTPγS. These authors did not preload the Rho protein with the nucleotide by EDTA treatment. It is feasible that the different assay conditions are responsible for these effects.

8 Possible Interactions of C3 Substrates with the Rhodopsin Receptor

The guanine nucleotide dependency of the C3-induced ADP-ribosylation of Rho is comparable with the ADP-ribosylation of G-proteins by pertussis toxin. Substrate of pertussis toxin is the inactive heterotrimeric G_i or transducin which has GDP bound, but not the activated and dissociated α-subunit of the G-protein which has GTP bound (Tsai et al. 1984; Van Dop et al. 1984; Ui 1990).

Therefore, stimulation of the light receptor rhodopsin, which causes the subsequent activation of transducin including GDP/GTP exchange and subunit dissociation, results in inhibition of pertussis toxin-catalyzed ADP-ribosylation. Recently, Wieland and coworkers (1990a) reported that C3 ADP-ribosylates low-molecular weight GTP-binding proteins in bovine retina. Light exposure apparently decreases the C3-catalyzed ADP-ribosylation of retinal 21-kDa proteins. Moreover, the apparent activation of the light receptor also decreased the ADP-ribosylation of exogenous RhoA protein, which was added to the incubation mixture (Wieland et al. 1990b). These findings were interpreted as indicating that the GTP-binding proteins which are substrates of C3 also interact with the rhodopsin receptor in the retina.

9 The Amino Acid Acceptor of C3-Induced ADP-Ribosylation

Recently, Sekine et al. (1989) showed that the *rho* protein is ADP-ribosylated at asparagine-41. Since all C3 substrates (RhoA, -B and -C; Rac 1 and 2) have asparagine at the same position, it is most likely that all these GTP-binding proteins are modified at the identical amino acid (Table 1). Asparagine is unique as an ADP-ribose receptor for the mono-ADP-ribosylation reaction catalyzed by C3. While cholera toxin (Moss and Vaughan 1978), C2 toxin (Vandekerckhove et al. 1988), and *C. perfringens* iota toxin ADP-ribosylate arginine (Vandekerckhove et al. 1987), pertussis toxin modifies cysteine residues (West et al. 1985). The acceptor for diphtheria toxin- and *P. aeruginosa* exotoxin A-catalyzed ADP-ribosylation is diphthamide, a posttranslationally modified

Table 1. Effector regions of low-molecular weight GTP-binding proteins

Protein	Effector region
c-Ha-Ras	27-HFVDE**YDPTIEDSY**RKQVV-45
c-Ki-Ras	27-HFVDE**YDPTIEDSY**RKQVV-45
c-N-Ras	27-HFVDE**YDPTIEDSY**RKQVV-45
Rap 1A	27-IFVEK**YDPTIEDSY**RKQVE-45
Rab 1	35-TYTES**YISTIGVDF**KIRTI-53
Ral	38-EFVED**YEPTKADSY**RKKVV-56
RhoA	29-QFPEV**YVPTVFENY**VADIE-47
RhoB	29-EFPEV**YVPTVFENY**VADIE-47
RhoC	29-QFPEV**YVPTVFENY**IADIE-47
RHO 1	34-QFPEV**YVPTVFENY**VADVE-52
RHO 2	31-KFPEQ**YHPTVFENY**VTDCR-49
Rac 1	27-AFPGE**YIPTVFDNY**SANVM-45
Rac 2	27-AFPGE**YIPTVFDNY**SANVM-45

The RhoA protein is ADP-ribosylated in asparagine-41. All GTP-binding proteins, which are putative substrates of C3 (RhoA, B, C; RHO 1 and RHO 2; Rac 1 and Rac 2) share asparagine in this position (underlined). By analogy with Ras proteins, asparagine-41 is located in the so-called effector region (boldface amino acids).

histidine (VAN NESS et al. 1980). The ADP-ribose-asparagine bond formed by C3 is particularly stable against hydroxylamine and sodium hydroxide (AKTORIES et al. 1988b). Whereas 0.5-*M* hydroxylamine cleaves the ADP-ribose bond formed by cholera or botulinum C2 toxin with a half-life of about 2 h, the C3-formed bond is stable. The ADP-ribose-asparagine bond is also stable toward mercury-(I)-salts (AKTORIES et al. 1988b), which split the pertussis toxin-formed cysteine bond of ADP-ribose (MEYER et al. 1988).

10 Effects of ADP-Ribosylation on GTP-Binding and GTPase Activity

In contrast to the effects of guanine nucleotides on the C3-induced ADP-ribosylation, various groups did not observe an influence of the ADP-ribosylation of Rho on nucleotide binding and/or GTPase activity of the Rho proteins purified from bovine or porcine brain or on the recombinant protein expressed in *E.coli* (BRAUN et al. 1989). Furthermore, the ADP-ribosylation reportedly does not affect the stimulation of the Rho GTPase by GAP (PATERSON et al. 1990). This finding is most surprising, because the ADP-ribose moiety is attached to Rho at asparagine-41 (SEKINE et al. 1989), which is located in a region analogous with the so-called effector region of Ras (PAI et al. 1989). In this area of Ras, the GAP protein is suggested to interact with the GTP-binding protein to stimulate GTP hydrolysis (ADARI et al. 1988). However, we observed recently that the steady state GTPase activity of recombinant RhoA is increased by ADP-ribosylation when RhoA protein was pretreated with C3 for only a short (10 min) period of time (unpublished observation). The reason for this discrepancy is not clear.

11 Functional Consequences of ADP-Ribosylation by C3

Our knowledge about the pathophysiological role of C3 and the functional consequences of the C3-induced ADP-ribosylation of GTP-binding proteins is still very limited. In general, these studies are hampered by the fact that C3 does not enter most cells. So far it is not clear whether C3 is a toxin or not. Injection of 100 μg of C3 into mice is apparently without obvious effects (unpublished observation). Thus, it has been suggested that C3 is a part of a holoenzyme, the binding component of which is not known at present. However, so far no evidence exists for an additional binding or transfer component. The problem of cell accessibility could be first by-passed by using the osmotic shock method to introduce C3 into cells (RUBIN et al. 1988). In NIH 3T3 cells, C3 induced rounding up of the cell body with formation of cell processes and occurrence of binucleated cells. The morphological changes were reversed after 2 days. In PC12 cells, C3 induced the formation of neurite-like processes. Recently, high concentrations of C3 (30–100 μg/ml) were shown to effect PC12 cells in a similar manner, inducing formation of neurite-like processes, growth inhibition, and induction of acetylcholine esterase activity (NISHIKI et al. 1990). Concomitantly, a 22-kDa protein was ADP-ribosylated. Further studies have been performed with Vero cells, which appear to be rather sensitive toward C3 (CHARDIN et al. 1989). Incubation with C3 causes rounding up of cells and ADP-ribosylation of about-21-kDa proteins. Furthermore, analysis of the cytoskeleton of treated cells shows a destruction of the microfilament network while the microtubule system is still intact. Similar effects are observed after treatment of rat hepatoma FAO cells with C3 (WIEGERS et al. 1991). Subsequent to alteration of the microfilaments of FAO cells, the intermediate filaments are redistributed, again without major alteration of the microtubule filaments. These studies were interpreted that the C3 substrates are somehow involved in the regulation of the cytoskeletal architecture, a view which has been corroborated by recent studies with the recombinant RhoA protein. In these studies a Rho mutant was used with valine instead of glycine in position 14, a mutation which renders the protein constitutively active by inhibition of the inherent GTPase activity. Microinjection of Val-14 RhoA into Swiss 3T3 cells induces rapid changes (15 min) in the cell morphology, with cell retraction and formation of spike-like processes (PATERSON et al. 1990). Thus the microinjection causes a phenotype completely different from that caused by injection of C3. Injection of normal Rho protein previously activated by GTPγS induces identical morphological changes. Interestingly, in contact-inhibited cells, which show no major actin filaments, the injection of Val-14 Rho protein induces the rapid formation of stress fibers. Prior ADP-ribosylation of the Rho protein by C3 prevents the morphological changes induced by Val-14 RhoA. On the other hand, microinjection of ADP-ribosylated normal RhoA induces effects similar to those observed after injection of C3. All these data suggested that the ADP-ribosylation of Rho renders the protein inactive (PATERSON et al. 1990).

A similar conclusion was drawn from studies with *X. laevis* oocytes (MOHR et al. 1990). *X. laevis* oocytes, which are normally arrested in the prophase of meiosis, can be triggered to complete meiosis by progesterone (MALLER and KREBS 1977). Microinjection of C3 into the oocytes causes induction of maturation and enhances the effects of progesterone on vesicle breakdown (RUBIN et al. 1988). In contrast, microinjection of Val-14 Rho into the oocytes induces a dramatic redistribution of the pigments from the animal pole. This effect is blocked by prior ADP-ribosylation of Val-14 Rho. As already mentioned, the Rho protein is ADP-ribosylated in asparagine-41, and, by analogy with Ras, the ADP-ribose acceptor amino acid appears to be located in the effector region (PAI et al. 1989). Provided that Ras and Rho proteins are sterically homologous, sterical hindrance in this area would be an explanation for the biological inactivation of Rho by ADP-ribosylation.

As mentioned above, the "small" GTP-binding proteins Rho and Rac are most probably posttranslationally modified by polyisoprenylation, as shown for Ras proteins. In *X. laevis* oocytes, lovastatin, which inhibits polyisoprenylation, inhibits the biological activity of Val-14 Rho (e.g., the induction of morphological changes). Therefore, it has been suggested that isoprenylation and membrane attachment is at least partially involved in the biological activation of Rho protein (MOHR et al. 1990).

12 *Clostridium limosum* ADP-Ribosyltransferase

Recent studies in our laboratory have shown that the ADP-ribosylation of low-mass GTP-binding proteins from the Rho/Rac family is not unique to *C. botulinum* C3 exoenzyme. A *C. limosum* strain isolated from a human lung abscess produces an ADP-ribosyltransferase which is closely related to C3 (JUST et al., submitted). The *C. limosum* enzyme has the same molecular mass as C3 and exhibits immunological cross-reactivity. The K_m of the *C. limosum* enzyme for NAD is 0.5–1 μM. The amino acid sequence analysis of various proteolytic peptides revealed an about 70% homology between the *C. limosum* enzyme and C3. Furthermore, the *C. limosum* enzyme is able to de-ADP-ribosylate Rho proteins previously modified by C3. These findings indicate that the novel enzymes not only ADP-ribosylate the same protein substrates but also modify Rho proteins in the identical amino acid. In contrast to C3, *C. limosum* exoenzyme is effectively auto-ADP-ribosylated in the presence of 0.01% SDS. Since the ADP-ribose incorporated by auto-ADP-ribosylation is as stable against hydroxylamine treatment as the ADP-ribose bond in Rho formed by C3, it is likely that the auto-ADP-ribosylation also occurs in asparagine (JUST et al., submitted).

13 Summary and Conclusions

C3 and C3-like ADP-ribosyltransferases modify the low-molecular-mass GTP-binding proteins Rho and Rac. ADP-ribosylation occurs in asparagine-41, which is located in the putative effector region of these highly conserved regulatory proteins. First studies indicate that the Rho proteins are somehow involved in the regulation of cytoskeletal proteins, e.g., microfilament proteins. Although the precise mechanism of the interaction of the C3 substrate with cytoskeletal elements is unclear, it appears that the ADP-ribosylation by C3 renders the GTP-binding protein biologically inactive. Thus C3 and/or C3-like ADP-ribosyltransferases may be useful instruments with which to study the physiological functions of its eukaryotic substrates. Moreover, those studies may help to elucidate whether these exoenzymes are of pathophysiological and pathogenetic relevance in diseases caused by clostridia producing these agents.

Acknowledgements. Studies reported herein and carried out in the laboratory of the authors were supported by the Deutsche Forschungsgemeinschaft (Ak 6/1–1, Ak 6/1–2) Sonderforschungsbereich 249 (A3), and the Fonds der Chemischen Industrie.

Notes added in proof: Recently, a C3-like endogenous ADP-ribosyltransferase from bovine brain has been described (Maehama et al. (1991) J Biol Chem 266: 10062–10065). Nemoto et al. (J Biol Chem 266: 19312–19319) reported on the *Clostridium botulinum* C3 ADP-ribosyltransferase gene showing a difference of about 40% between the cDNA reported by Popoff et al. (1990). The poly-isoprenylation of Rho (Katayama et al. (1991) J Biol Chem 266: 12639–12645; Hori et al. (1991) Oncogene 6: 515–522) and Rac (Kinsella et al. (1991) J Biol Chem 266: 9786–9794) has been studied in detail. Diekmann et al. (Nature (1991) 351: 400–402) reported that the Rho–GAP protein reveals high homology with the product of the *bcr* (break point cluster region) gene, the translocation breakpoint in Philadelphia chromosome-positive chronic myeloid leukaemias. Recently, it has been shown that the activation of the NADPH oxidase involves the rac1 protein (A. Abo et al. (1991) Nature 353: 668–670).

References

Adam-Vizi V, Rösener S, Aktories K, Knight DE (1988) Botulinum toxin-induced ADP-ribosylation and inhibition of exocytosis are unrelated events. FEBS Lett 238: 277–280

Adari H, Lowy DR, Willumsen BM, der Channing J, McCormick F (1988) Guanosine triphosphate activating protein (GAP) interacts with the p21 *ras* effector binding domain. Science 240: 518–521

Aktories K, Frevert J (1987) ADP-ribosylation of a 21–24 kDa eukaryotic protein(s) by C3, a novel botulinum ADP-ribosyltransferase, is regulated by guanine nucleotide. Biochem J 247: 363–368

Aktories K, Bärmann M, Ohishi I, Tsuyama S, Jakobs KH, Habermann E (1986a) Botulinum C2 toxin ADP-ribosylates actin. Nature 322: 390–392

Aktories K, Ankenbauer T, Schering B, Jakobs KH (1986b) ADP-ribosylation of platelet actin by botulinum C2 toxin. Eur J Biochem 161: 155–162

Aktories K, Weller U, Chhatwal GS (1987) *Clostridium botulinum* type C produces a novel ADP-ribosyltransferase distinct from botulinum C2 toxin. FEBS Lett 212: 109–113

Aktories K, Rösener S, Blaschke U, Chhatwal GS (1988a) Botulinum ADP-ribosyltransferase C3. Purification of the enzyme and characterization of the ADP-ribosylation reaction in platelet membranes. Eur J Biochem 172: 445–450

Aktories K, Just I, Rosenthal W (1988b) Different types of ADP-ribose protein bonds formed by botulinum C2 toxin, botulinum ADP-ribosyltransferase C3 and pertussis toxin. Biochem Res Commun 156: 361–367

Aktories K, Braun U, Rösener S, Just I, Hall A (1989) The *rho* gene product expressed in *E. coli* is a substrate of botulinum ADP-ribosyltransferase C3. Biochem Biophys Res Commun 158: 209–213

Avraham H (1990) *rho* gene amplification and malignant transformation. Biochem Biophys Res Commun 168: 114–124

Avraham H, Weinberg RA (1989) Characterization and expression of the human *rho*H12 gene product. Mol Cell Biol 9: 2058–2066

Barbacid M (1987) *ras* Genes. Ann Rev Biochem 56: 779–827

Banga HS, Gupta SK, Feinstein MB (1988) Botulinum toxin D ADP-ribosylates a 22–24 kDa membrane protein in platelets and HL-60 cells that is distinct from $p21^{N-ras}$. Biochem Biophys Res Commun 155: 263–269

Bokoch GM, Katada T, Northup JK, Hewlett EL, Gilman AG (1983) Identification of the predominant substrate for ADP-ribosylation by islet activating protein. J Biol Chem 258: 2072–2075

Bokoch GM, Parkos CA, Mumby SM (1988) Purification and characterization of the 22 000-dalton GTP-binding protein substrate for ADP-ribosylation by botulinum toxin, G_{22k}. J Biol Chem 263: 16744–16749

Bourne HR, Sanders DA, McCormick F (1991) The GTPase superfamily: conserved structure and molecular mechanism. Nature 349: 117–127

Braun U, Habermann B, Just I, Aktories K, Vandekerckhove J (1989) Purification of the 22 kDa protein substrate of botulinum ADP-ribosyltransferase C3 from procine brain cytosol and its characterization as a GTP-binding protein highly homologus to the *rho* gene product. FEBS Lett 243: 70–76

Cassel D, Pfeuffer T (1978) Mechanism of cholera toxin action: covalent modification of the guanyl nucleotide-binding protein of the adenylate cyclase system. Proc Natl Acad Sci USA 75: 2669–2673

Chardin P, Tavitian A, (1986) The *ral* gene: a new *ras*-related gene isolated by the use of a synthetic probe. EMBO J 5: 2203–2208

Chardin P, Madaule P, Tavitian A (1988) Coding sequence of human *rho* cDNAs clone 6 and clone 9. Nucleic Acids Res 16: 2717

Chardin P, Boquet P, Madaule P, Popoff MR, Rubin EJ, Gill DM (1989) The mammalian G protein *rho*C is ADP-ribosylated by *Clostridium botulinum* exoenzyme C3 and affects actin microfilament in Vero cells. EMBO J 8: 1087–1092

Collier RJ (1990) Diphtheria toxin: structure and function of a cytocidal protein. In: Moss J, Vaughan M (eds) ADP-ribosylating toxins and G proteins. American Society For Microbiology, Washington, pp 3–19

De Vos AM, Tong L, Milburn MV, Matias PM, Jancarik J, Noguchi S, Nishimura S, Miura K, Ohtsuka E, Kim S (1988) Three-dimensional structure of an oncogenic protein: catalytic domain of human c-H-*ras*. Science 239: 888–893

Didsbury J, Weber RF, Bokoch GM, Evans T, Snyderman R (1989) rac, a novel *ras*-related family of proteins that are botulinum toxin substrates. J Biol Chem 264: 16378–16382

Didsbury JR, Uhling RJ, Syndermann R (1990) Isoprenylation of the low molecular mass GTP-binding proteins *rac* 1 and *rac* 2: possible role in membrane localization. Biochem Biophys Res Commun 171: 804–812

Downward J, Riehl R, Wu L, Weinberg RA (1990) Identification of a nucleotide exchange-promoting activity for $p21^{ras}$. Proc Natl Acad Sci USA 87: 5998–6002

Eklund MW, Poysky FT (1972) Activation of a toxic component of *Clostridium botulinum* type C and D by trypsin. Appl Microbiol 24: 108–113

Eklund MW, Poysky FT, Reed SM (1972) Bacteriophage and the toxigenicity of *Clostridium botulinum* type D. Nature, New Biology 235: 16–17

Garrett MD, Self AJ, von Oers C, Hall A (1989) Identification of distinct cytoplasmic targets for *ras*, R-*ras* and *rho* regulatory proteins. J Biol Chem 264: 10–13

Gibbs JB, Schaber MD, Allard WJ, Sigal IS, Scolnick EM (1988) Purification of *ras* GTPase activating protein from bovine brain. Proc Natl Sci USA 85: 5026–5030

Habermann B, Mohr C, Just I, Aktories K (1991) ADP-ribosylation and de-ADP-ribosylation of the *rho* protein by *Clostridium botulinum* exoenzyme C3. Regulation by EDTA, guanine nucleotides and pH. Biochim Biophys Acta 1077, 253–258

Habermann E, Dreyer F (1986) Clostridial neurotoxins: handling and action at the cellular and molecular level. Curr Top Microbiol Immunol 129: 93–179

Hall A (1990) The cellular functions of small GTP-binding proteins. Science 249: 635–640

Hancock JF, Magee AI, Childs JE, Marshall CJ (1989) All *ras* proteins are polyisoprenylated but only some are palmitoylated. Cell 57: 1167–1177

Hoshijima M, Kondo J, Kikuchi A, Yamamoto K, Takai Y (1990) Purification and characterization from bovine brain membranes of a GTP-binding protein with a M_r of 21 000 ADP-ribosylated by an ADP-ribosyltransferase contaminated in botulinum toxin type C1-identification as the *rho*A gene product. Mol Brain Res 7: 9–16

Honjo T, Nishizuka Y, Hayaishi O, Kato I (1968) Diphtheria-toxin-dependent-adenosine diphosphate ribosylation of aminoacyl transferase II and inhibition of protein synthesis. J Biol Chem 243: 3553–3555

Iglewski BH, Kabat D (1975) NAD-dependent inhibition of protein synthesis by *Pseudomonas aeruginosa* toxin. Proc Natl Acad Sci USA 72: 2284–2289

Isomura M, Kaibuchi K, Yamamoto T, Kawamura S, Katayama M, Takai Y (1990) Partial purification and characterization of GDP dissociation stimulator (GDS) for the *rho* proteins from bovine brain cytosol. Biochem Biophys Res Commun 169: 652–659

Kikuchi A, Yamamoto K, Fujita T, Takai Y (1988) ADP-ribosylation of the bovine brain *rho* protein by botulinum toxin type C1. J Biol Chem 263: 16303–16308

Madaule P, Axel R (1985) A novel *ras*-related gene family. Cell 41: 31–40

Madaule P, Axel R, Myers AM (1987) Characterization of two members of the *rho* gene family from the yeast *Saccharomyces cerevisiae*. Proc Natl Acad Sci USA 84: 779–783

Maller JL, Krebs EG (1977) Progesterone-stimulated meiotic cell divison in *Xenopus* oocytes. J Biol Chem 252: 1712–1718

Matsuoka I, Syuto B, Kurihara K, Kubo S (1987) ADP-ribosylation of specific membrane proteins in pheochromocytoma and primary-cultured brain cells by botulinum neurotoxins type C and D. FEBS Lett 216: 295–299

Matsuoka I, Sakuma H, Syuto B, Moriishi K, Kubo S, Kurihara K (1989) ADP-ribosylation of 24–26-kDa GTP-binding proteins localized in neuronal and non-neuronal cells by botulinum neurotoxin D. J Biol Chem 264: 706–712

Mege JL, Volpi M, Becker EL, Sha'afi RJ (1988) Effect of botulinum D toxin on neutrophils. Biochem Biophys Res Commun 152: 926–932

Meyer T, Koch R, Fanick W, Hilz H (1988) ADP-ribosyl proteins formed by pertussis toxin are specifically cleaved by mercury ions. Biol Chem Hoppe Seyler 369: 579–583

Mohr C, Just I, Hall A, Aktories K (1990) Morphological alterations of *Xenopus* oocytes induced by valine-14 $p21^{rho}$ depend on isoprenylation and are inhibited by *Clostridium botulinum* C3 ADP-ribosyltransferase. FEBS Lett 275: 168–172

Morii N, Sekine A, Ohashi Y, Nakao K, Imura H, Fujiwara M, Narumiya S (1988) Purification and properties of the cytosolic substrate for botulinum ADP-ribosyltransferase. J Biol Chem 263: 12420–12426

Moriishi K, Syuto B, Oguma K, Saito M (1990) Separation of toxic activity and ADP-ribosylation activity of botulinum neurotoxin D. J Biol Chem 265: 16614–16616

Moss J, Vaughan M (1977) Mechanism of action of choleragen. Evidence for ADP-ribosyltransferase activity with arginine as an acceptor. J Biol Chem 252: 2455–2457

Narumiya S, Sekine A, Fujiwara M (1988) Substrate for botulinum ADP-ribosyltransferase, Gb, has an amino acid sequence homologous to a putative *rho* gene product. J Biol Chem 263: 17255–17257

Nishiki T, Narumiya S, Morii N, Yamamoto M, Fujiwara M, Kamata Y, Sakaguchi G, Kozaki S (1990) ADP-ribosylation of the *rho*/*rac* proteins induces growth inhibition, neurite outgrowth and acetylcholine esterase in cultures PC-12 cells. Biochem Biophys Res Commun 167: 265–272

Ohashi Y, Narumiya S (1987) ADP-ribosylation of a M_r 21 000 membrane protein by type D botulinum toxin. J Biol Chem 262: 1430–1433

Pai EF, Kabsch W, Krengel U, Holmes KC, John J, Wittinghofer A (1989) Structure of the guanine-nucleotide-binding of the Ha-*ras* oncogene product p21 in the triphosphate conformation. Nature 341: 209–214

Paterson HF, Self AJ, Garrett MD, Just I, Aktories K, Hall A (1990) Microinjection of recombinant p21-*rho* induces rapid change in cell morphology. J Cell Biol 111: 1001–1007

Pfeuffer T, Helmreich EJM (1988) Structural and functional relationship of guanosine triphosphate binding proteins. Curr Top Cell Regul 29: 129–216

Pizon V, Chardin P, Lerosey I, Olofson B, Tavitian A (1988) Human cDNA *rap* 1 and *rap* 2 homologous to the Drosophila gene *Dras 3* encode proteins closely related to *ras* in the "effector" region region. Oncogene 3: 201–204

Polakis PG, Weber RF, Nevins B, Didsbury JR, Evans T, Synderman R (1989) Identification of the *ral* and *rac1* gene products, low molecular mass GTP-binding proteins from human platelets. J Biol Chem 264: 16383–16389

Popoff MR, Boquet P (1988) *Clostridium spiroforme* toxin is a binary toxin which ADP-ribosylates cellular actin. Biochem Biophys Res Commun 152: 1361–1368

Popoff M, Boquet P, Gill DM, Eklund MW (1990) DNA sequence of exoenzyme C3, an ADP-ribosyltransferase encoded by *Clostridium botulinum* C and D phages. Nucleic Acids Res 18: 1291

Quilliam LA, Brown JH, Buss JE (1988) A 22-kDa *ras*-related G-protein is the substrate for an ADP-ribosyltransferase from *Clostridium botulinum*. FEBS Lett 238: 22–26

Rösener S, Chhatwal GS, Aktories K (1987) Botulinum ADP-ribosyltransferase C3 but not botulinum neurotoxins C1 and D ADP-ribosylates low molecular mass GTP-binding proteins. FEBS Lett 224: 38–42

Rubin EJ, Gill DM, Boquet P, Popoff MR (1988) Functional modification of a 21-kilodalton G protein when ADP-ribosylated by exoenzyme C3 of *Clostridium botulinum*. Mol Cell Biol 8: 418–426

Schering B, Bärmann M, Chhatwal GS, Geipel U, Aktories K (1988) ADP-ribosylation of skeletal muscle and non-muscle actin by *Clostridium perfringens* iota toxin. Eur J Biochem 171: 225–229

Sekine A, Fujiwara M, Narumiya S (1989) Asparagine residue in the *rho* gene product is the modification site for botulinum ADP-ribosyltransferase. J Biol Chem 264: 8602–8605

Toki C, Oda K, Ikehara Y (1989) Demonstration of GTP-binding proteins and ADP-ribosylated proteins in rat liver golgi fraction. Biochem Biophys Res Commun 164: 333–338

Touchot N, Chardin P, Tavitian A (1987) Four additional members of the *ras* gene superfamily isolated by an oligonucleotide strategy: molecular cloning of YPT-related cDNAs from a rat brain library. Proc Natl Acad Sci USA 84: 8210–8214

Trahey M, McCormick F (1987) A cytoplasmic protein stimulates normal N-*ras* p21 GTPase, but does not affect oncogenic mutants. Science 238: 542–545

Tsai SC, Adamik R, Kanaho Y, Hewlett EL, Moss J (1984) Effect of guanyl nucleotides and rhodopsin on ADP-ribosylation of the inhibitory GTP-binding component of adenylate cyclase by pertussis toxin. J Biol Chem 259: 15320–15323

Ueda T, Kikuchi A, Ohga N, Yamamoto J, Takai Y (1990) Purification and characterization from bovine brain cytosol of a novel regulatory protein inhibiting the dissociation of GDP from and the subsequent binding of GTP to *rho*B p20, a *ras* p21-like GTP-binding protein. J Biol Chem 265: 9373–9380

Ui M (1990) Pertussis toxin as a valuable probe for G-protein involvement in signal transducin. In: Moss J, Vaughan M (eds) ADP-ribosylating toxins and G proteins. American Society for Microbiology, Washington, pp 45–77

Vandekerckhove J, Schering B, Bärmann M, Aktories K (1987) *Clostridium perfringens* iota toxin ADP-ribosylates skeletal muscle actin in Arg-177. FEBS Lett 225: 48–52

Vandekerckhove J, Schering B, Bärmann M, Aktories K (1988) Botulinum C2 toxin ADP-ribosylates cytoplasmic β-/γ-actin in arginine 177. J Biol Chem 263: 696–700

Van Dop C, Yamanaka G, Steinberg F, Sekura RD, Manclark CR, Stryer L, Bourne HR (1984) ADP-ribosylation of transducin by pertussis toxin blocks the light-stimulated hydrolysis of GTP and cGMP in retinal photoreceptors. J Biol Chem 259: 23–26

Van Ness BG, Howard JB, Bodley JW (1980) ADP-ribosylation of elongation factor 2 by diphtheria toxin. NMR spectra and proposed structures of ribosyldiphthamide and its hydrolysis products. J Biol Chem 255: 10710–10716

West RE, Moss J, Vaughan M, Liu T, Liu TY (1985) Pertussis toxin-catalyzed ADP-ribosylation of transducin. J Biol Chem 260: 14428–14430

Wick MJ, Iglewski BH (1990) *Pseudomonas aeruginosa* exotoxin A. In: Moss J, Vaughan M (eds) ADP-ribosylating toxins and G proteins. American Society for Microbiology, Washington, pp 31–43

Wiegers W, Just I, Müller H, Traub P, Aktories K (1991) Alteration of the cytoskeleton of mammalian cells cultured in vitro by *Clostridium botulinum* C2 toxin and C3 ADP-ribosyltransferase. Eur J Cell Biol 54: 237–245

Wieland T, Ulibarri I, Aktories K, Gierschik P, Jakobs KH (1990a) Interaction of small G proteins with photoexcited rhodopsin. FEBS Lett 263: 195–198

Wieland T, Ulibarri I, Gierschik P, Aktories K, Jakobs KH (1990b) Interaction of recombinant *rho*A GTP-binding proteins with photoexcited rhodopsin. FEBS Lett 274: 111–114

Williamson KC, Smith LA, Moss J, Vaughan M (1990) Guanine nucleotide-dependent ADP-ribosylation of soluble *rho* catalyzed by *Clostridium botulinum* C3 ADP-ribosyltransferase. J Biol Chem 265: 20807–20812

Wolfman A, Macara IG (1990) A cytosolic protein catalyzes the release of GDP from $p21^{ras}$. Science 248: 67–69

Yamamoto J, Kikuchi A, Ueda T, Ohga N, Takai Y (1990) A GTPase-activating protein for *rho*B p20, a *ras* p21-like GTP-binding protein—partial purification, characterization and subcellular distribution in rat brain. Mol Brains Res 8: 105–111

Yeramian P, Chardin P, Madaule P, Tavitian A (1987) Nucleotide sequence of human *rho* cDNA clone 12. Nucleic Acids Res 15: 1869

Pseudomonas aeruginosa Exoenzyme S

J. COBURN

1 Introduction

Pseudomonas aeruginosa is an opportunistic pathogen that secretes a number of potential virulence factors. Two of these, exotoxin A and exoenzyme S, catalyze the transfer of the ADP-ribose moiety of NAD to proteins in eukaryotic cells. Exotoxin A catalyzes the ADP-ribosylation of elongation factor 2 (EF-2), leading to disruption of protein synthesis. It has been well characterized and is reviewed elsewhere in this volume. Exoenzyme S has been less thoroughly studied, but several lines of evidence suggest that it might play a role in pathogenesis. In preliminary experiments exoenzyme S appeared to be unselective in choice of substrate proteins, but recent work has shown that it preferentially ADP-ribosylates several of the low-molecular weight GTP-binding proteins. Furthermore, like cholera toxin, exoenzyme S requires a eukaryotic protein for enzymic activity.

Department of Molecular Biology and Microbiology, Tufts University School of Medicine, 136 Harrison Avenue, Boston, MA 02111, USA

Present address: Division of Rheumatology and Immunology, New England Medical Center, Box 406, 750 Washington St., Boston, MA 02111 USA

Current Topics in Microbiology and Immunology, Vol. 175

2 Initial Characterization of Exoenzyme S

Exoenzyme S is an ADP-ribosyltransferase secreted by many strains *P. aeruginosa*. It was first discovered because some *P. aeruginosa* culture supernatant fluids catalyzed the transfer of far more ADP-ribose than could be accounted for by the ADP-ribosylation of the EF-2 available by the already known exotoxin A. Closer examination of these culture supernatants revealed the presence of a second ADP-ribosyltransferase, which was named exoenzyme S (IGLEWSKI et al. 1978). Exoenzyme S catalyzes the transfer of only the ADP-ribose portion of NAD to numerous proteins in crude wheat germ extracts, but does not modify nucleic acids (IGLEWISKI et al. 1978). Digestion of the reaction product with snake venom phosphodiesterase released only AMP, demonstrating that exoenzyme S catalyzes a mono-ADP-ribosylation (IGLEWSKI et al. 1978). In contrast to exotoxin A, exoenzyme S does not modify EF-2, is relatively stable to heat, and is sensitive to treatment with urea (IGLEWSKI et al. 1978). Polyclonal antisera to exotoxin A do not neutralize exoenzyme S activity or form a precipitate with exoenzyme S in immunodiffusion assays (IGLEWSKI et al. 1978). Finally, exoenzyme S activity is maximal at pH 6–6.5 and is relatively insensitive to ethylenediaminetetracetate (EDTA), sodium azide, and salt concentration in that pH range (THOMPSON et al. 1980). Exoenzyme S activity is also insensitive to dithiothreitol (DTT), which stimulates the enzymic activity of exotoxin A.

Culture conditions have been established which maximize the production of exoenzyme S. In flask cultures, the medium which allows maximal exoenzyme S yields is similar to that used for exotoxin A production; it includes dialyzed trypticase soy broth, monosodium glutamate, glycerol, and a chelating agent (THOMPSON et al. 1980). The chelating agent is required for production of exoenzyme S, but not for production of exotoxin A. Another difference is that while exotoxin A synthesis appears to be iron-regulated, exoenzyme S synthesis does not (THOMPSON et al. 1980). Further coditions for maximal exoenzyme S production in flask cultures include growth at 32 °C and vigorous aeration. We have established conditions for production of exoenzyme S in a 20-liter fermentor. The requirements include dilution of a culture grown in rich medium into a minimal medium containing M9 salts, succinate, and 30-m*M* EDTA, and growth at 30 °C with tight aeration control (COBURN et al. 1991). Thus production of exoenzyme S, like that of many other potential virulence factors from many different bacteria, appears to be tightly regulated and maximal when the growth conditions are less than optimal.

Exoenzyme S is secreted into the medium in two forms: M_r 53 000 and M_r 49 000 (IGLEWSKI 1988). The two forms appear to be related: they are immunologically cross-reactive, antisera prepared against both forms neutralize activity, and the two proteins yield common peptides after digestion with trypsin, chymotrypsin, and cyanogen bromide (IGLEWSKI 1988). When the total protein content of culture supernatant fluids were examined, the levels of the two forms of exoenzyme S increased or decreased in parallel, depending on growth conditions. The 49000- and 53000-Da forms of the enzyme share the same amino-terminal amino acid sequences (IGLEWSKI, personal communication; our unpublished results), and transposon-insertion mutants which are deficient in exoenzyme S production do not secrete either form (IGLEWSKI 1988). The 49000-Da form is enzymically active, but the 53000-Da form is not, and neither one is toxic when injected into mice (NICAS and IGLEWSKI 1985) or when artificially introduced into fibroblasts in culture (our unpublished results). The 53000-Da form may therefore be a precursor of the 49000-Da form, which is enzymically active only after a 4000-Da peptide is removed, presumably from the carboxyl terminus. Activation by proteolysis appears to be a common feature of bacterial toxins, including tetanus and botulinum neurotoxins (MIDDLEBROOK and DORLAND 1984) and shigella toxin (OLSNES et al. 1981). Other bacterial ADP-ribosyltransferases that are activated by limited proteolysis include diphtheria toxin (DRAZIN et al. 1971) *P. aeruginosa* exotoxin A (VASIL et al. 1977), and cholera toxin (MEKALANOS et al. 1979). An alternative, but less likely, possibility is that the two forms of exoenzyme S are products of two distinct genes. If so, they would have to be encoded in the same transcription unit or regulon, given the transposon insertion results. The two forms might then differ in their target cell or substrate specificities.

When exoenzyme S was first reported, it was only the third bacterial enzyme demonstrated to be an ADP-ribosyltransferase (although three phage ADP-ribosylating enzymes had been identified). Thus the phenomenon of ADP-ribosylation as a common mechanism among bacterial toxins had not yet been recognized. The addition of exoenzyme S to the list contributed to the idea of that ADP-ribosylation might be an important way for pathogenic bacteria to damage host cells and stimulated the search for ADP-ribosylation as a mechanism used by other bacterial toxins.

3 Preliminary Identification of Exoenzyme S Substrates

Although exoenzyme S appeared to ADP-ribosylate many proteins, we found that a number of these can be accounted for by the intermediate filament protein vimentin and its fragments (COBURN et al. 1989a). Vimentin is a very abundant cellular protein that serves as a relatively poor substrate for exoenzyme S, yet may account for a large proportion of the total [^{32}P]ADP-ribose incorporation when exoenzyme S and [^{32}P]NAD are added to cell lysates. Fragments of vimentin, which are generated by a specific cellular calcium-activated protease and which cannot be incorporated into filaments, are better substrates for exoenzyme S than is the intact protein. In addition, filamentous vimentin is a poorer substrate than is dissociated vimentin. Finally, ADP-ribosylated vimentin did not appear to reassociate to form filaments. Therefore, although vimentin appears to be a relatively poor substrate, exoenzyme S in vivo may have an effect on the cytoskeleton through disruption of vimentin polymerization.

3.1 The Preferred Substrates Are GTP-Binding Proteins

As the family of bacterial ADP-ribosyltransferases expanded, it became apparent that many of these enzymes preferentially modify GTP-binding proteins in eukaryotic cells. These include diphtheria toxin and *P. aeruginosa* exotoxin A, which modify the same residue of EF-2 (HONJO et al. 1968; IGLEWSKI and KABAT 1975); cholera toxin, which modifies $G_{s\alpha}$ (GILL and MEREN 1978), pertussis toxin, which ADP-ribosylates $G_{i\alpha}$ (MURAYAMA and UI 1983); and *Clostridium botulinum* exoenzyme C3, which ADP-ribosylates the Rho proteins (RUBIN et al. 1988; BRAUN et al. 1989; CHARDIN et al. 1989). The cytoskeletal protein actin had also been identified as a substrate for several other clostridial toxins (AKTORIES et al. 1986; VANDEKERCKHOVE et al. 1987; POPOFF et al. 1988; POPOFF and BOQUET 1988). Although vimentin and other abundant proteins account for a large proportion of the total ADP-ribosylation catalyzed by exoenzyme S, we found that, like many of the bacterial ADP-ribosyltransferases, exoenzyme S preferentially ADP-ribosylates GTP-binding proteins (COBURN et al. 1989b). The preferred exoenzyme S substrates comprise a subset of the low-molecular weight GTP-binding proteins and include the H-*ras* and K-*ras* gene products (reviewed by SANTOS and NEBREDA 1989). These proteins are ADP-ribosylated at lower exoenzyme S concentrations than are other proteins even though they are much less abundant than many of the other exoenzyme S substrates. In addition, ADP-ribosylation of this group of proteins saturates within the range of exoenzyme S concentrations tested, while modification of other proteins continues to increase with increasing exoenzyme S concentrations (COBURN et al. 1989b). These results reflect not only the low abundance of the preferred substrates, but also the limited number of modification sites on each protein. In fact, we have several lines of evidence that indicate that each substrate molecule is modified at only one site (COBURN et al. 1989a, b).

ADP-ribosylations catalyzed by other bacterial ADP-ribosyltransferases result in changes in the functions of the GTP-binding protein substrates, but ADP-ribosylation catalyzed by exoenzyme S did not alter GTP binding, GTP for GDP exchange, or GTP hydrolysis by $p21^{ras}$ (our published results). Furhermore, no change was observed in $p21^{ras}$ interaction with guanine nucleotide release factor (GRF) (WOLFMAN and MACARA 1990), the protein that stimulates release of GDP from $p21^{ras}$, or interaction with GTPase-activating protein (GAP) (TRAHEY and MCCORMICK 1987), the protein that stimulates the GTP hydrolysis activity of $p21^{ras}$ (our unpublished observations). ADP-ribosylation of $p21^{ras}$ by exoenzyme S did, however, cause a substantially larger shift in electrophoretic mobility than would be expected from the addition of the ADP-ribose group. This result suggests that a significant change in the conformation of the $p21^{ras}$ protein might occur upon ADP-ribosylation by exoenzyme S. If such a conformational change does occur, the ADP-ribosylation of p21^{ras} might alter its interaction with cellular proteins aside from GRF and GAP, whose existence is implied by numerous studies on the function of p21^{ras}, but not proved. Despite intensive study, the cellular functions of p21^{ras} and many of the related proteins remain a mystery. If exoenzyme S does modify the functions of its substrates, it may prove useful as a tool to explore the functions of the proteins of the *ras* superfamily.

3.1.1 Exoenzyme S Requires A Eukaryotic Protein for Activity

In order to identify specific low molecular weight GTP-binding proteins as substrates for exoenzyme S, we attempted to ADP-ribosylate candidate proteins which had been partially purified from *Escherichia coli* cells expressing their cloned genes. However, although p21^{ras} was a substrate in eukaryotic cell lysates, the protein expressed in *E. coli* was not a substrate, although it was present and active as determined by other criteria. As it is well-known that the ADP-ribosyltransferase activity of cholera toxin is stimulated by the eukaryotic protein ADP-ribosylation factor (ARF) (KHAN and GILMAN 1986; GILL and COBURN 1987), we tested whether exoenzyme S has a similar requirement. We found that *exoenzyme S was able to ADP-ribosylate p21^{ras}* made in *E. coli* only if lysates of eukaryotic cells were added to the in vitro reaction. The cellular factor that allows the ADP-ribosylation reaction to proceed is absolutely required for ADP-ribosylation of p21^{ras} and all other substrates by exoenzyme S (COBURN et al. 1991). The factor which allows exoenzyme S activity is sensitive to trypsin and elutes in the macromolecular fraction when chromatographed through Sephadex G-50. The active protein has a molecular weight of approximately 29 000 Da and a pI of 4.3–4.5. Activity is found in all eukaryotic cells and tissues but is absent from all bacterial species tested to date. We (COBURN et al. 1991) have named this protein factor activating exoenzyme S (FAS).

3.2 Other Preferred Exoenzyme S Substrates

By adding exoenzyme S, NAD, and FAS to proteins partially purified from lysates of *E. coli*, we were able to ADP-ribosylate some, but not all, of the *ras*-related GTP-binding proteins. We found that Rap1A (PIZON et al. 1988), Ral (CHARDIN and TAVITIAN 1986), Rab 3 and Rab 4 (TOUCHOT et al. 1987) were all ADP-ribosylated by exoenzyme S. The Rho (MADAULE and AXEL 1985) and Rab 1 (TOUCHOT et al. 1987) proteins, G_p (EVANS et al. 1986), and ARF (KAHN and GILMAN 1986; GILL and COBURN 1987) were not substrates for exoenzyme S. Based on comparisons of the sequences of the proteins which are ADP-ribosylated and those which were not, in addition to the lack of effect of ADP-ribosylation on GTP handling by p21^{ras} and the observation that exoenzyme S modifies arginine residues (COBURN et al. 1989b), we predict that the ADP-ribosylation site is arginine-123 of p21^{ras}. Analysis of the crystal structure of p21^{ras} predicts that arginine-123 is located on an outer surface loop of the protein (JURNAK et al. 1990). The function of this portion of the protein has not yet been defined or even thoroughly tested, but the addition of a fairly large acidic group such as ADP-ribose to the surface of a protein might be expected to alter the cellular interactions of that protein. For example, ADP-ribosylation of $G_{i\alpha}$ by pertussis toxin disrupts interaction of Gi with receptors (MIDDLEBROOK and DORLAND 1984), and ADP-ribosylation of EF-2 by diphtheria toxin or *P. aeruginosa* exotoxin A prevents functional interaction of EF-2 with the ribosome (COLLIER 1975).

4 The Role of Exoenzyme S in Pathogenesis

Several lines of evidence suggest that exoenzyme S plays a role in *P. aeruginosa* infections, although the evidence is indirect. After transposon mutagenesis of *P. aeruginosa* strains which produce exoenzyme S, derivatives were selected which no longer produced either form of exoenzyme S, but otherwise appeared to be identical to the parental strains (NICAS and IGLEWSKI 1984; WOODS and SOKOL 1985). The exoenzyme S mutants (S^-) were then compared with the parental strains in two animal model systems. In the burned mouse model, the LD_{50} for the parental strain was 30 CFU, while that of the S^- derivative was at least 1.6×10^5 CFU (NICAS and IGLEWSKI 1985; NICAS et al. 1985a). The S^- mutant established infection at the site of inoculation as well as did the parental strain, but spread to other sites much less efficiently. When both strains were inoculated together, both disseminated efficiently, suggesting that exoenzyme S might be important in overcoming host defenses against spread from the site of infection, rather than for survival after dissemination (NICAS and IGLEWSKI 1985). Furthermore, anti-exoenzyme S antibodies protected burned mice aganist disseminating infection after inoculation with an exoenzyme S-producing strain of *P. aeruginosa* (NICAS and IGLEWSKI 1985). In the rat lung infection model, little or no histological change was apparent after infection with the S^- mutant, while the parental strain produced widespread, large areas of damage to pulmonary tissue (NICAS and IGLEWSKI 1985; NICAS et al. 1985b). The transposon itself did not interfere with dissemination, since another mutant, which produced exoenzyme S but was auxotrophic for leucine, was as virulent as the parental strain. Similar results have been obtained using a different strain of *P. aeruginosa* and a different transposon (WOODS and SOKOL 1985), but in both of these systems it was possible that the transposons had disrupted one or more genes required for exoenzyme S production, but not the structural gene encoding exoenzyme S itself. Although the only gross changes in the culture supernatants of the transposon mutants were the lack of exoenzyme S activity and cross-reactive material, the transposons might in fact have damaged other genes, with more pleiotropic effects.

Another series of experiments has tested the effects of purified exoenzyme S on cultured cells and in animal models. The purified exoenzyme S used in these studies has been reported to be toxic to cells and mice (WOODS and QUE 1987), results which conflict with those obtained in other laboratories (NICAS and IGLEWSKI 1985; our unpublished results). In further experiments, the same group shows that exoenzyme S causes gross damage to pulmonary tissue after intratracheal administration (WOODS et al. 1988). The material used for these in vivo experiments, however, was not enzymically active and thus has not been definitively identified as exoenzyme S (WOODS and QUE 1987). In addition, the purified material differs in several characteristics (including molecular weight and solubility) from exoenzyme S as originally described. Furthermore the *P. aeruginosa* strain which was used in these studies, DGI, differs in several ways from 388, the strain which was used in all other work. The recent molecular cloning of the gene encoding the material used (SOKOL et al. 1990) may allow some of these problems to be resolved. However, when expressed, the cloned gene does not produce enzymically active exoenzyme S in *E. coli*, but does in a *P. aeruginosa* strain which already produces the inactive 53000-DA form of exoenzyme S. Thus there is a strong possibility that the cloned DNA may not contain the structural gene for exoenzyme S, but instead contains a gene encoding a factor required for production of the active 49000-Da species, or even a third ADP-ribosyltransferase. In fact, the *P. aeruginosa* leukocidin (or cytotoxin), which has already been cloned and sequenced (HAYASHI et al. 1989), has recently been identified as an ADP-ribosyltransferase (NODA et al. 1990). Therefore, while the possibilities that the gene encoding exoenzyme S has been cloned and that exoenzyme S is in some form toxic to cultured cells and to animals cannot be ruled out, rigorous proof is lacking. An intriguing possibility is that the enzymically active form of exoenzyme S is not toxic to cells. The active 49000-Da species might lack a functional cell-binding epitope which, when present, inhibits ADP-ribosyltransferase activity. Many of the other bacterial ADP-ribosyltransferases have distinct cell-binding and enzymically active domains, and require some sort of processing for enzymic activity.

There are several other, less direct indications that exoenzyme S plays a role in pathogenesis. At least 40% of the strains isolated from human infections produce enzymically active exoenzyme S and at least 90% of both clinical and environmental isolates produce cross-reactive material (IGLEWSKI 1988). Preliminary screening of clinical isolates indicated that increased mortality due to *P. aeruginosa* infection was correlated with exoenzyme S, but not with exotoxin A production (THOMPSON et al. 1980). A later study of many more clinical isolates showed that a higher rate of mortality in patients with systemic *P. aeruginosa* infections was associated with strains that produce both exotoxin A and exoenzyme S than with strains that produce either ADP-ribosyltransferase alone (SOKOL et al. 1981). Additional evidence supporting a role for exoenzyme S in pathogenesis was obtained in an animal model for *P. aeruginosa* infection. When burned mice were infected with a *P. aeruginosa* strain which produces high levels of exoenzyme S but little exotoxin A, exoenzyme S activity was present in the serum before the bacteria were detectable and was found in extracts of skin from the site of inoculation (BJORN et al. 1979). Thus exoenzyme S is produced in vivo, at least in the experimental model, an important prerequisite for considering the possible role of exoenzyme S in pathogenesis.

5 Conclusion

The secretion of two distinct ADP-ribosyltransferases by *P. aeruginosa* suggests that the enzymes play very different roles in pathogenesis. The substrate profiles and differential toxicities indicate that the two enzymes might have distinct target cells or species preferences. Exotoxin A disrupts protein synthesis by ADP-ribosylating EF-2, killing the host cell. In contrast, exoenzyme S preferentially ADP-ribosylates several low-molecular weight GTP-binding proteins of the *ras* gene superfamily. Several of these GTP-binding proteins have been shown to have roles in trafficking of vesicles through the exocytic and endocytic pathways of eukaryotic cells (CHAVRIER et al. 1990; GOUD et al. 1988; MELANCON et al. 1987; SALMINEN and NOVICK 1987). Thus, exoenzyme S might disrupt normal trafficking of vesicles in the affected cell. Exoenzyme S might interfere with secretion of granules from cells of the host defense system (e.g., neutrophils) or disrupt the normal phagocytic function of macrophages. It has been proposed that exoenzyme S might interfere with the host defense system at the site of infection (NICAS and IGLEWSKI 1985; IGLEWSKI 1988), and ADP-ribosylation of low-molecular weight GTP-binding proteins in neutrophils and macrophages might destroy their antimicrobial activities, allowing the spread of the exoenzyme S-producing strains of *P. aeruginosa*. These ideas are far from proven, but they are consistent with the evidence that exoenzyme S contributes to the efficiency of dissemination of *P. aeruginosa* in infection (NICAS and IGLEWSKI 1985). It is also possible that the ADP-ribosylation of vimentin might also damage the cell by disrupting the cytoskeleton. We have seen modification of only a small proportion of the total vimentin, but if vimentin is only available as a substrate when monomeric the ADP-ribosylation might have an effect on the cytoskeleton in the long term. An alternative view is that exoenzyme S might contribute to the survival of *P. aeruginosa* in the natural environment. More than 90% of environmental isolates of *P. aeruginosa* produce exoenzyme S, as detected using anti-exoenzyme S antibodies (NICAS et al. 1985b; IGLEWSKI 1988). In addition, exoenzyme S has considerably higher in vitro enzymic activity at 25 °C than at 37 °C. Therefore, the role of exoenzyme S might be due to damage eukaryotic soil and water microorganisms, plants, or cold-blooded animals. Exoenzyme S is not likely to be involved in killing other bacteria in the environment, since FAS activity appears to be present only in eukaryotes.

The precise role of exoenzyme S in pathogenesis or in the survival of *P. aeruginosa* in the environment will probably become clearer during the next few years. A clone of the gene encoding exoenzyme S, as originally defined, would allow several questions to be addressed. These include the most basic questions: Is exoenzyme S a toxin? Is the enzymically active protein capable of binding to and entering eukaryotic cells, or is a distinct cell-binding component encoded elsewhere on the chromosome? Does the 53000-Da form represent a precursor of the 49000-Da protein, or are they the products of different genes? How is production of exoenzyme S regulated, and is it coordinately regulated with other virulence determinants? Another series of experiments might lead to a better understanding of the mechanism by which exoenzyme S contributes to pathogenesis. Does exoenzyme S actively impair host defenses? What effect does ADP-ribosylation catalyzed by exoenzyme S have on the functions of the GTP-binding protein substrates? How do these effects, If any, affect the normal functions of the target cells? The answers to all these questions will contribute to our understanding of the role of exoenzyme S in the pathogenesis of *P. aeruginosa* infections.

Acknowledgements. This chapter was made possible by work done in the laboratory of D. Michael Gill, and by his enthusiasm for research. Unfortunately, Dr. Gill died suddenly in June of 1990. The author would like to thank B. H. Iglewski, A. L. Sonenshein, and A. Donohue-Rolfe for critical review of the manuscript.

References

Aktories K, Barmann M, Ohishi I, Tsuyma S, Jakobs KH, Habermann E (1986) Botulinum C2 toxin ADP-ribosylates actin. Nature 322: 390

Bjorn MJ, Pavlovskis OR, Thompson MR, Iglewski BH (1979) Production of exoenzyme S during *Pseudomonas aeruginosa* infections in burned mice. Infect Immun 24: 837–842

Braun U, Habermann B, Just I, Aktories K, Vandekerckhove J (1989) Purification of the 22-kDa protein substrate of botulinum ADP-ribosyltransferase C3 from porcine brain cytosol and its characterization as a GTP-binding protein highly homologous to the *rho* gene product. FEBS Lett 243: 70–76

Chardin P, Tavitian A (1986) The *ral* gene: a new *ras* related gene isolated by the use of a synthetic probe. EMBO J 5: 2203–2208

Chardin P, Boquet P, Madaule P, Popoff MR, Rubin EJ, Gill DM (1989) The mammalian G protein *rho*C is ADP-ribosylated by *Colstridium botulinum* exoenzyme C3 and affects actin microfilaments in Vero cells. EMBO J 8: 1087–1092

Chavrier P, Parton RG, Hauri HP, Simons K, Zerial M (1990) Localization of low molecular weight GTP-binding proteins to exocytic and entocytic compartments. Cell 62: 317–329

Coburn J, Dillon ST, Iglewski BH, Gill DM (1989a) Exoenzyme S of *Pseudomonas aeruginosa* ADP-ribosylates the intermediate filament protein vimentin. Infect Immun 57: 996–998

Coburn J, Wyatt RT, Iglewski BH, Gill Dm (1989b) Several GTP-binding proteins, including $p21^{cHras}$, are preferred substrates of *Pseudomonas aeruginosa* exoenzyme S. J Biol Chem 264: 9004–9008

Coburn J, Kane AV, Feig L, Gill DM (1991) *Pseudomonas aeruginosa* exoenzyme S requires a eukaryotic protein for ADP-ribosyl transferase activity. J Biol Chem 266: 6438–6446

Collier RJ (1975) Diphtheria toxin: mode of action and structure. Bacteriol Rev 39: 54–85

Drazin R, Kandel J, Collier RJ (1971) Structure and activity of diphtheria toxin: attack by trypsin at a specific site within the intact molecule. J Biol Chem 246: 1504–1510

Evans T, Brown ML, Fraser ED, Northup JK (1986) Purification of the major GTP-binding proteins from human placental membranes. J Biol Chem 261: 7052–7059

Gill DM, Coburn J (1987) ADP-ribosylation by cholera toxin: functional analysis of a cellular system that stimulates the enzymic activity of cholera toxin fragment A1. Biochemistry 26: 6364–6371

Gill DM, Meren R (1978) ADP-ribosylation of membrane proteins catalyzed by cholera toxin: basis of the activation of adenylate cyclase. Proc Natl Acad Sci USA 75: 3050–3054

Goud B, Salminen A, Walworth NC, Novick PJ (1988) A GTP-binding protein required for secretion rapidly associates with secretory vesicles and the plasma membrane in yeast. Cell 53: 753–768

Hayashi T, Kamio Y, Hishinuma F, Usami Y, Titani K, Terawaki Y (1989) *Pseudomonas aeruginosa* cytotoxin: the nucleotide sequence of the gene and the mechanism of activation of the protoxin. Mol Microbiol 3: 861–868

Honjo T, Nishizuka Y, Hayaishi O (1968) Diphtheria toxin-dependent adenosine ribosylation of aminoacyl transferase II and inhibition of protein synthesis. J Biol Chem 243: 3553–3555

Iglewski BH (1988) Pseudomonas toxins. In: Hardegree MC, Tu AT (eds) Handbook of toxins, vol. 4. Dekker, New York, pp 249–265

Iglewski BH, Kabat D (1975) NAD-dependent inhibition of protein synthesis by *Pseudomonas aeruginosa* toxin. Proc Natl Acad Sci USA 72: 2284–2288

Iglewski BH, Sadoff J, Bjorn MJ, Maxwell ES (1978) *Pseudomonas aeruginosa* exoenzyme S: an adenosine diphospate ribosyltransferase distinct from toxin A. Proc Natl Acad Sci USA 75: 3211–3215

Jurnak F, Heffron S, Bergmann E (1990) Conformational changes involved in the activation of *ras* p21: implications for related proteins. Cell 60: 525–528

Kahn RA, Gilman AG (1986) The protein cofactor necessary for ADP-ribosylation of Gs by cholera toxin is itself a GTP binding protein. J Biol Chem 261: 7906–7911

Madaule P, Axel R (1985) A novel *ras* related gene family. Cell 41: 31–40

Mekalanos JJ, Collier RJ, Roming WR (1979) Enzymic activity of cholera toxin: relationships to proteolytic processing, disulfide bond reduction, and subunit composition. J Biol Chem 254: 5855–5861

Melancon P, Glick BS, Malhotra V, Weidman PJ, Serafini T, Gleason ML, Orci L, Rothman JE (1987) Involvement of GTP binding "G" proteins in transport through the Golgi stack. Cell 51: 1053–1062

Middlebrook JL, Dorland RB (1984) Bacterial toxins: cellular mechanisms of action. Microbiol Rev 48: 199–221

Murayama T, Ui M (1983) Loss of the inhibitory function of the guanine nucleotide regulatory component of adenylate cyclase due to its ADP ribosylation by islet-activating protein, pertussis toxin, in adipocyte membranes. J Biol Chem 258: 3319–3326

Nicas TI, Iglewski BH (1984) Isolation and characterization of transposon-induced mutants of *Pseudomonas aeruginosa* deficient in production of exoenzyme S. Infect Immun 45: 470–474

Nicas TI, Iglewski BH (1985) Contribution of exoenzyme S to the virulence of *Pesudomonas aeruginosa*. Antibiot Chemother 36: 40–48

Nicas TI, Bradley J, Lochner JE, Iglewski (1985a) The role of exoenzyme S in infections with *Pseudomonas aeruginosa*. J Infect Dis 152: 716–721

Nicas TI, Frank DW, Stenzel P, Lile JD, Iglewski BH (1985b) Role of exoenzyme S in chronic *Pseudomonas aeruginosa* lung infections. Eur J Clin Microbiol 4: 175–179

Noda M, Kato I, Wang X, Hirayama T (1990) ADP-ribosylation and activation of PI-specific phospholipase C by Pseudomonal leukocidin (Abstr) In: Basic research and clinical aspects of *Pseudomonas aeruginosa* infection 3rd International Symposium, Tokyo

Olsnes S, Reisbig R, Eiklid K (1981) Subunit structure of Shigella cytotoxin. J Biol Chem 256: 8732–8738

Pizon V, Chardin P, Lerosey I, Oloffsson B, Tavitian A (1988) Human cDNAs rap1 and rap2 homologous to the *Drosophila* gene Dras3 encode proteins closely related to *ras* in the "effector" region. Oncogene 3: 201–204

Popoff MR, Boquet P (1988) *Clostridium spiroforme* toxin is a binary toxin which ADP-ribosylates cellular actin. Biochem Biophys Res Commun 152: 1361–1368

Popoff MR, Rubin EJ, Gill DM, Boquet P (1988) Actin-specific ADP-ribosyltransferase produced by a *Clostridium difficile* strain. Infect Immun 56: 2229–2306

Rubin EJ, Gill DM, Boquet P, Popoff MR (1988) Functional modification of a 21-kilodalton G protein when ADP-ribosylated by exoenzyme C3 of *Clostridium botulinum*. Mol Cell Biol 8: 418–426

Salminen A, Novick PJ (1987) A *ras*-like protein is required for a post-Golgi event in yeast secretion. Cell 49: 5527–5538

Santos E, Nebreda AR (1989) Structural and functional properties of *ras* proteins. FASEB J 3: 2151–2163

Sokol PA, Iglewski BH, Hager TA, Sadoff JC, Cross AS, McManus A, Farber BF, Iglewski WJ (1981) Production of exoenzyme S by clinical isolates of *Pseudomonas aeruginosa*. Infect Immun 34: 147–153

Sokol PA, Dennis JJ, MacDougall PC, Sexton M, Woods DE (1990) Cloning and expression of the *Pseudomonas aeruginosa* exoenzyme S toxin gene. Microb Pathog 8: 243–257

Thompson MR, Bjorn MJ, Sokol PA, Lile JD, Iglewski BH (1980) Exoenzyme S: an ADP-ribosyl transferase produced by *Pseudomonas aeruginosa*. In: Smulson M, Sugimura T (eds) Novel ADP-ribosylations of regulatory enzymes and proteins. Elsevier, Amsterdam, pp 425–432

Touchot N, Chardin P, Tavitian A (1987) Four additional members of the *ras* gene superfamily isolated by an oligonucleotide strategy: molecular cloning of YPT-related cDNAs from a rat brain library. Proc Natl Acad Sci USA 84: 8210–8214

Trahey M, McCormick F (1987) A cytoplasmatic protein stimulates normal N-*ras* p21 GTPase, but does not affect oncogenic mutants. Science 238: 542–545

Vandekerckhove J, Schering B, Barmann M, Aktories K (1987) *Clostridium perfringens* iota toxin ADP-ribosylates skeletal muscle actin in Arg-177. FEBS Lett 225: 48–52

Vasil ML, Kabat D, Iglewski BH (1977) Structure-activity relationships of an exotoxin of *Pseudomonas aeruginosa*. Infect Immun 16: 353–361

Wolfman A, Macara IG (1990) A cytosolic protein catalyzes the release of GDP from $p21^{ras}$. Science 248: 67–69

Woods DE, Hwang WS, Shahrabadi MS, Que JU (1988) Alteration of plumonary structure by *Pseudomonas aeruginosa* exoenzyme S. J Med Microbiol 26: 133–141

Woods DE, Que JU (1987) Purification of *Pseudomonas aeruginosa* exoenzyme S. Infect Immun 55: 579–586

Woods DE, Schaffer MS, Rabin HR, Campbell GD, Sokol PA (1986) Phenotypic comparison of *Pseudomonas aeruginosa* strains isolated from a variety of sources. J Clin Microbiol 24: 260–264

Woods DE, Sokol PA (1985) Use of transposon mutants to assess the role of exoenzyme S chronic pulmonary disease due to *Pseudomonas aeruginosa*. Eur J Clin Microbiol 4: 163–169

Subject Index

Current Topics in Microbiology and Immunology

Volumes published since 1986 (and still available)

Vol. 131: **Doerfler, Walter; Böhm, Petra (Ed.):** The Molecular Biology of Baculoviruses. 1986. 44 figs. VIII, 169 pp. ISBN 3-540-17073-1

Vol. 132: **Melchers, Fritz; Potter, Michael (Ed.):** Mechanisms in B-Cell Neoplasia. Workshop at the National Cancer, Institute, National Institutes of Health, Bethesda, MD, USA, March 24–26, 1986. 1986. 156 figs. XII, 374 pp. ISBN 3-540-17048-0

Vol. 133: **Oldstone, Michael B. (Ed.):** Arenaviruses. Genes, Proteins, and Expression. 1987. 39 figs. VII, 116 pp. ISBN 3-540-17246-7

Vol. 134: **Oldstone, Michael B. (Ed.):** Arenaviruses. Biology and Imminotherapy. 1987. 33 figs. VII, 242 pp. ISBN 3-540-14322-6

Vol. 135: **Paige, Christopher J.; Gisler, Roland H. (Ed.):** Differentiation of B Lymphocytes. 1987. 25 figs. IX, 150 pp. ISBN 3-540-17470-2

Vol. 136: **Hobom, Gerd; Rott, Rudolf (Ed.):** The Molecular Biology of Bacterial Virus Systems. 1988. 20 figs. VII, 90 pp. ISBN 3-540-18513-5

Vol. 137: **Mock, Beverly; Potter, Michael (Ed.):** Genetics of Immunological Diseases. 1988. 88 figs. XI, 335 pp. ISBN 3-540-19253-0

Vol. 138: **Goebel, Werner (Ed.):** Intracellular Bacteria. 1988. 18 figs. IX, 179 pp. ISBN 3-540-50001-4

Vol. 139: **Clarke, Adrienne E.; Wilson, Ian A. (Ed.):** Carbohydrate-Protein Interaction. 1988. 35 figs. IX, 152 pp. ISBN 3-540-19378-2

Vol. 140: **Podack, Eckhard R. (Ed.):** Cytotoxic Effector Mechanisms. 1989. 24 figs. VIII, 126 pp. ISBN 3-540-50057-X

Vol. 141: **Potter, Michael; Melchers, Fritz (Ed.):** Mechanisms in B-Cell Neoplasia 1988. Workshop at the National Cancer Institute, National Institutes of Health, Bethesda, MD, USA, March 23–25, 1988. 1988. 122 figs. XIV, 340 pp. ISBN 3-540-50212-2

Vol. 142: **Schüpach, Jörg:** Human Retrovirology. Facts and Concepts. 1989. 24 figs. 115 pp. ISBN 3-540-50455-9

Vol. 143: **Haase, Ashley T.; Oldstone Michael B. A. (Ed.):** In Situ Hybridization 1989. 22 figs. XII, 90 pp. ISBN 3-540-50761-2

Vol. 144: **Knippers, Rolf; Levine, A. J. (Ed.):** Transforming. Proteins of DNA Tumor Viruses. 1989. 85 figs. XIV, 300 pp. ISBN 3-540-50909-7

Vol. 145: **Oldstone, Michael B. A. (Ed.):** Molecular Mimicry. Cross-Reactivity between Microbes and Host Proteins as a Cause of Autoimmunity. 1989. 28 figs. VII, 141 pp. ISBN 3-540-50929-1

Vol. 146: **Mestecky, Jiri; McGhee, Jerry (Ed.):** New Strategies for Oral Immunization. International Symposium at the University of Alabama at Birmingham and Molecular Engineering Associates, Inc. Birmingham, AL, USA, March 21–22, 1988. 1989. 22 figs. IX, 237 pp. ISBN 3-540-50841-4

Vol. 147: **Vogt, Peter K. (Ed.):** Oncogenes. Selected Reviews. 1989. 8 figs. VII, 172 pp. ISBN 3-540-51050-8

Vol. 148: **Vogt, Peter K. (Ed.):** Oncogenes and Retroviruses. Selected Reviews. 1989. XII, 134 pp. ISBN 3-540-51051-6

Vol. 149: **Shen-Ong, Grace L. C.; Potter, Michael; Copeland, Neal G. (Ed.):** Mechanisms in Myeloid Tumorigenesis. Workshop at the National Cancer Institute, National Institutes of Health, Bethesda, MD, USA, March 22, 1988. 1989. 42 figs. X, 172 pp. ISBN 3-540-50968-2

Vol. 150: **Jann, Klaus; Jann, Barbara (Ed.):** Bacterial Capsules. 1989. 33 figs. XII, 176 pp. ISBN 3-540-51049-4

Vol. 151: **Jann, Klaus; Jann, Barbara (Ed.):** Bacterial Adhesins. 1990. 23 figs. XII, 192 pp. ISBN 3-540-51052-4

Vol. 152: **Bosma, Melvin J.; Phillips, Robert A.; Schuler, Walter (Ed.):** The Scid Mouse. Characterization and Potential Uses. EMBO Workshop held at the Basel Institute for Immunology, Basel, Switzerland, February 20–22, 1989. 1989. 72 figs. XII, 263 pp. ISBN 3-540-51512-7

Vol. 153: **Lambris, John D. (Ed.):** The Third Component of Complement. Chemistry and Biology. 1989. 38 figs. X, 251 pp. ISBN 3-540-51513-5

Vol. 154: **McDougall, James K. (Ed.):** Cytomegaloviruses. 1990. 58 figs. IX, 286 pp. ISBN 3-540-51514-3

Vol. 155: **Kaufmann, Stefan H. E. (Ed.):** T-Cell Paradigms in Parasitic and Bacterial Infections. 1990. 24 figs. IX, 162 pp. ISBN 3-540-51515-1

Vol. 156: **Dyrberg, Thomas (Ed.):** The Role of Viruses and the Immune System in Diabetes Mellitus. 1990. 15 figs. XI, 142 pp. ISBN 3-540-51918-1

Vol. 157: **Swanstrom, Ronald; Vogt, Peter K. (Ed.):** Retroviruses. Strategies of Replication. 1990. 40 figs. XII, 260 pp. ISBN 3-540-51895-9

Vol. 158: **Muzyczka, Nicholas (Ed.):** Viral Expression Vectors. 1992. 20 figs. IX, 176 pp. ISBN 3-540-52431-2

Vol. 159: **Gray, David; Sprent, Jonathan (Ed.):** Immunological Memory. 1990. 38 figs. XII, 156 pp. ISBN 3-540-51921-1

Vol. 160: **Oldstone, Michael B. A.; Koprowski, Hilary (Ed.):** Retrovirus Infections of the Nervous System. 1990. 16 figs. XII, 176 pp. ISBN 3-540-51939-4

Vol. 161: **Racaniello, Vincent R. (Ed.):** Picornaviruses. 1990. 12 figs. X, 194 pp. ISBN 3-540-52429-0

Vol. 162: **Roy, Polly; Gorman, Barry M. (Ed.):** Bluetongue Viruses. 1990. 37 figs. X, 200 pp. ISBN 3-540-51922-X

Vol. 163: **Turner, Peter C.; Moyer, Richard W. (Ed.):** Poxviruses. 1990. 23 figs. X, 210 pp. ISBN 3-540-52430-4

Vol. 164: **Bækkeskov, Steinnun; Hansen, Bruno (Ed.):** Human Diabetes. 1990. 9 figs. X, 198 pp. ISBN 3-540-52652-8

Vol. 165: **Bothwell, Mark (Ed.):** Neuronal Growth Factors. 1991. 14 figs. IX, 173 pp. ISBN 3-540-52654-4

Vol. 166: **Potter, Michael; Melchers, Fritz (Ed.):** Mechanisms in B-Cell Neoplasia 1990. 143 figs. XIX, 380 pp. ISBN 3-540-52886-5

Vol. 167: **Kaufmann, Stefan H. E. (Ed.):** Heat Shock Proteins and Immune Response. 1991. 18 figs. IX, 214 pp. ISBN 3-540-52857-1

Vol. 168: **Mason, William S.; Seeger, Christoph (Ed.):** Hepadnaviruses. Molecular Biology and Pathogenesis. 1991. 21 figs. X, 206 pp. ISBN 3-540-53060-6

Vol. 169: **Kolakofsky, Daniel (Ed.):** Bunyaviridae. 1991. 34 figs. X, 256 pp. ISBN 3-540-53061-4

Vol. 170: **Compans, Richard W. (Ed.):** Protein Traffic in Eukaryotic Cells. Selected Reviews. 1991. 14 figs. X, 186 pp. ISBN 3-540-53631-0

Vol. 171: **Kung, Hsing-Jien; Vogt, Peter K. (Eds.):** Retroviral Insertion and Oncogene Activation. 1991. 18 figs. X, 179 pp. ISBN 3-540-53857-7

Vol. 172: **Chesebro, Bruce W. (Ed.):** Transmissible Spongiform Encephalopathies. 1991. 48 figs. X, 288 pp. ISBN 3-540-53883-6

Vol. 173: **Pfeffer, Klaus; Heeg, Klaus; Wagner, Hermann; Riethmüller, Gert (Ed.):** Function and Specificity of γ/δ T Cells. 1991. 41 figs. XII, 296 pp. ISBN 3-540-53781-3

Vol. 174: **Fleischer, Bernhard; Sjögren, Hans Olov (Eds.):** Superantigens. 1991. 13 figs. IX, 137 pp. ISBN 3-540-54205-1